The Dentist's Guide to Sleep Apnea Implementation

Your Step-by-Step Guide to a Comprehensive Sleep Program

Meghna Dassani DMD

First printing 2021

ISBN: ISBN: 978-1-7366589-5-6 (Paperback)

Soapbox Publishing

3083 W. Antelope View Dr.

Garden City ID 83714

www.meghnadassani.com

Dedication

For Nandini and Maadhvi.

My reasons for being, every minute of every day.

Table of Contents

Introduction – What Sleep Dentistry Has Done for Me and My Practice

I've always prided myself on being a hard worker. I worked hard in school and built a dental practice in Mumbai when I was in my early 20s. I moved to the US to be able to grow...my family and more, earned my DMD from BU, and in 2011 I started building my current practice in Houston. I was constantly focused on improving my clinical skills, growing my practice, becoming bigger and better in every way. There was just one problem.

My two beautiful daughters were growing up without a mother focused on their needs. Family and friends on two continents were having personal crises and health crises and I couldn't be fully present for them. I love dentistry, but I also love the people in my life, and I needed a way to balance my practice and personal life while also making the world a better place.

Sleep dentistry has allowed me to do this. I am helping patients like never before, by addressing root causes and creating real cures. My team is on fire because they know that the work they do really matters and they see how happy and healthy our patients have become. Best of all, my practice is more profitable, so I am able to reduce my clinical days as well.

Now, I really do have it all. I have a practice that energizes me and helps make the world a better place. I have time to connect and be present to my friends and family around the world. And, most of all, I have time to enjoy my family, especially as my girls grow into teens and just need more attention, conversation, and fun times with their parents.

Sleep Dentistry was the missing piece to balance my life as a dedicated, focused clinician and my life as a caring mom, daughter, sister, and friend. It can do the same for you: Save lives, energize your practice, and allow you to be there for your family.

If you're trying to decide whether you want to make the transition to sleep dentistry, or if you've taken any courses and need a handy reference, this book is for you. It won't replace a sleep seminar, but it can give you the basic nuts and bolts of implementing sleep dentistry in your practice. As you read, you'll notice that there's an "Implementation on Target" section at the end of each chapter. These are goals for you and your practice as you prepare to launch your sleep dentistry program.

Sleep dentistry has been an amazing addition to my practice and my life. I want to help you make it an amazing addition to yours!

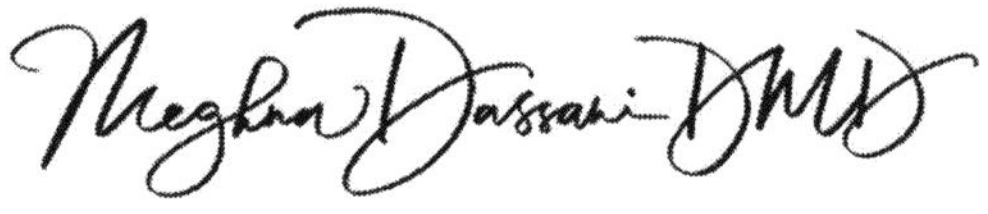

Part I: Becoming a Sleep Breathing Evangelist

How do you become a Sleep Dentist with a thriving practice? Before you can understand the how of implementing sleep dentistry, you need to understand the why. Why are we doing this? Why is this an incredibly important service to offer our patients and communities? Why is the struggle of changing the focus of your practice worth the work and time?

The first step is to learn about sleep and why it's important. Sleep medicine isn't something you can add to your practice grudgingly. Once you understand how important good sleep is to our bodies, our brains, our moods, and our lives, you'll want your family, friends, and patients to learn about sleep. And once you see how sleep-disordered breathing (SDB) can destroy families, livelihoods, and lives, you'll be passionate about identifying and treating it in your practice.

1: How Sleep Builds Our Brains and Bodies

In this chapter, you'll find:

- A quick review of sleep stages
- A brief summary of the benefits of sleep.

If you'd like to dig deeper, try my book, ***Airway is Life,*** or read ***Why We Sleep*** by Matthew Walker, Ph.D.

I was starting to get a little depressed about my patients' health. I saw the same people year after year, and it just seemed like they were in decline. Even patients my age just kept adding new health problems to the list. Their teeth and gums were affected, of course, but it was pretty obvious that dental problems were a symptom of the disease process, not the cause.

Sometimes, sleep seems almost like a punishment. You're a busy person with things to do! You have new things to learn, chores to catch up on, kids to care for, a practice you want to grow, and what about fun? Shouldn't you have some time to relax? Instead, each and every night, you have to stop everything you're doing and go to sleep, or you'll pay for it later.

It's no wonder toddlers fight sleep. Sleep is stopping. Sleep is boring. Sleep is nothing, just a pause, right? Wrong. Sleep is what keeps us healthy, happy and human. We need sleep to function at our best. When college students pull all-nighters or busy moms stay up late binge-watching Netflix, they may think that they're using their time efficiently.

In reality, they're crippling their mind and body. You need sleep almost as much as you need food. Good sleep restores you, solidifies new learning, and protects your body from damage. There's a reason the Geneva Convention lists sleep deprivation as a form of torture.

To implement sleep medicine in your dental practice, you're going to need a decent understanding of what sleep is and how healthy sleep makes healthy people. If you've already attended my course or read my book *Airway is Life*, a lot of this will be review for you. Otherwise, get ready for a whirlwind tour through Sleep 101.

What Sleep Looks Like to A Scientist

Sleep science is a fairly new field. We didn't really have the tools to study sleep until the mid-twentieth century. By 1957, we'd learned that there are 5 stages of sleep, divided into NREM and REM. The brain moves through all these stages during the night, and our body needs all five stages to remain healthy.

Stage 0: When You're Awake

When you're awake, your brain waves, heart rate, breathing, and body temperature are constantly in flux. You're looking around, responding to the world, speeding up and slowing down, and constantly changing. You're taking in and processing information, eating and processing food, and moving around constantly. The only constant is change.

NREM Stage 1: Drifting Off

After a long day, you finally have a chance to lie down. You sink into your pillow and close your eyes. Within a few minutes, your breathing and heart rate slow. Your body temperature begins to drop. Your brainwaves change too. They become lower voltage than your daytime signals, and their pattern begins to change.

In Stage 1, your thoughts become more random and confused. You stop understanding the conversations and sounds around you. If someone wakes you up, you may not remember having slept at all.

In stage one, you may experience "sleep jerks," where you feel like you're falling or thrashing and jerk yourself awake.

Most people spend between 1 and 7 minutes in this stage of light sleep. For example, when an exhausted new parent takes catnaps where they drift off for a few minutes in the middle of work or chores, they're hitting this stage of sleep. After you've spent several minutes in Stage 1 NREM, your brainwaves change again, and you've entered Stage 2.

Stage 2 NREM: Light Sleep

In Stage 2 NREM, your brainwaves start forming "sleep spindles." If someone wakes you during Stage 2, you've only been in a light sleep. You can wake up and feel refreshed even though you haven't completed a complete sleep cycle. Many '"power naps'" take advantage of a short period of Stage 2 sleep.

You'll remain in this stage for ten to twenty-five minutes. Slowly, the sleep spindles will become fewer, and the brain waves take on the slow, rhythmic patterns that mean that you've slipped into a deeper sleep.

Stages 3 and 4 NREM: Deep Sleep

Some scientists distinguish between Stage 3 and Stage 4 NREM, while others say that they're both parts of the same deep sleep. During these stages, a healthy person experiences slow, regular breathing, a slow heart rate, and synchronized, slow delta brain waves. This is the sleep you need to feel really and truly rested.

If you're a parent, you've probably seen a baby or child in a deep sleep. This is when they go limp. You can lift their arm, and it just falls back into place. You can move them around from a car to a bed, and they never even stir. Deeply sleeping adults can be hard to wake too, but their brains are still open to environmental stimuli. Researchers have found that during brief periods during each brain wave, the brain can respond to outside noises. So, even when you are deeply asleep, you can still hear the strange crash outside, the crying child, or the smoke alarm. Your brain is designed to keep you safe, even when you're sleeping.

This stage usually lasts from 20-40 minutes. It ends with a return to Stage 2 for 5-10 minutes. After revisiting Stage 2, you don't return to Stage 1. Instead, you enter a state called REM.

REM: The Dreaming State

In REM, or rapid eye movement sleep, your brain is as active as when you're awake. Sometimes it's even more active. Your eyes move rapidly, but the rest of your body experiences a kind of paralysis, so you won't move around and hurt yourself while you are dreaming. The rational centers of your brain are suppressed, but your emotional centers are running the show. The amount of time you spend in REM depends on the sleep cycle you're in. At the beginning of the night, your periods of REM are very short. Then, as the night goes on and you complete more sleep cycles, you spend more and more time in REM.

Sleep Cycles

Your brain moves between Stage 2, deep sleep, and REM sleep all night long. Over the course of a good night's sleep, you'll spend about half the time in Stage 2. In each 90-minute period, you'll experience Stage 2, Stages 3 and 4, and REM sleep. About 4 hours into your sleep, you may wake up and briefly move around, use the bathroom, or get a drink of water. Then you'll start back at Stage 1 and begin again.

Hypnograms

A hypnogram is a diagram showing when a sleeper is in each stage and how long they spend there. Sleep specialists can study hypnograms to detect problems in someone's sleep. For instance, a lack of deep sleep or too much REM too early in the night can help diagnose a sleep disorder.

STAGES OF **SLEEP**

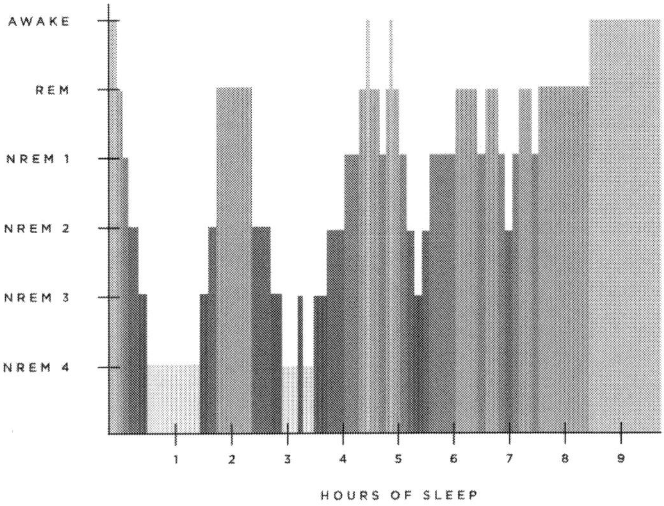

Hypnograms are also useful for educating your team and patients about healthy sleep and how our brain moves between stages of sleep.

I had a good rapport with my patients, and I wanted to help them. They were all seeing multiple specialists who never talked to each other. Their health problems were being treated in isolation, but there was something bigger going on. I just wasn't sure what I, as a dentist, could do to help, and it was frustrating.

What Healthy Sleep Does for the Brain, Body, and Moods

Why are scientists so interested in sleep? Because the more we learn about it, the more important it gets. We're constantly finding out about new ways that sleep protects our bodies and our brains. For instance, many researchers who study autism spectrum disorders are realizing that, at the root, some kids with ASD may have underlying sleep issues that cause or exacerbate their symptoms. We're finding sleep links with mental illnesses as well. And many physical issues may have their roots in bad sleep. It's impossible to give a comprehensive list of everything sleep does for your brain and body. What follows is a quick list to jog your memory and help you educate your team and patients.

Sleep Regulates Hormones

Bodies aren't built to be "on" 24-7. They need a period of sleep each day to reset, restore, and renew. Some of the hormones sleep regulates include:

- **Human Growth Hormone** - HGH is released during slow-wave sleep early in the night. In children, it helps them grow bigger. In adults, it causes the body to repair and replace damaged cells, it breaks down fat for energy, and it helps the body build muscle. When someone is trying to lose weight but staying up late, they're reducing the effectiveness of HGH and making their goals harder to reach.
- **Cortisol** - Cortisol is the stress hormone. The body suppresses it during sleep so that all of the body's systems get a break from 'fight or flight.'
- **Ghrelin** - Ghrelin is the hormone that makes people feel hungry. When someone sleeps well, it's suppressed. Good sleep means no midnight snack cravings.
- **Leptin** - Leptin is the hormone that promotes feelings of satiety. It's increased during sleep so that the sleeper feels full and burns calories.

The following chart sums up the hormonal action of sleep. Keep it handy for talking to your patients and team members!

HORMONE	WITH SLEEP	WITHOUT SLEEP
Human Growth Hormone (HGH)	Increases Sends signal to body to grow and heal	No increase Body continues to take damage because you are awake Repair process doesn't occur Over time, more and more damage, harder to reverse
Cortisol (Stress Hormone)	Decreases Break from stress Rest from fight or flight Reduced damage and inflammation and pain	Doesn't decrease, may increase More stress More time in fight or flight More inflammation More damage to every system of your body
Ghrelin (Hunger Hormone)	Decreases You don't crave food while you sleep You do burn calories in sleep	Continues to increase at intervals Get hungry every few hours Eat extra meals and calories Weight gain
Leptin (Satiety Hormone)	Increases You feel full and satisfied Your body is told it's OK to use calories	Decreases You crave food Your body tries to store more calories as fat Your body burns fewer calories, to conserve fat Weight Gain

Sleep and Learning

Sleep is essential for learning. During the day, all the senses take in information, we think about it, and we try to learn new things. Sleep is when the brain consolidates our learning so that we can use it later. There are a few different ways in which sleep helps us learn:

- **Clearing out the short-term memory** - Our short-term memory is based in the hypothalamus. This part of the brain only has a limited amount of storage space, like a photo card in a camera. When it gets full, we literally can't learn anymore. This is why small children need naps. Everything is new to them, so their hypothalamus runs out of space quickly. This is also why students studying for a big test will feel like their brain is literally full. They need a burst of NREM sleep to keep learning. This process can happen pretty quickly, which is why a power nap can often wake up an overwhelmed brain.

- **Storing new knowledge where it can be retrieved** - Slow-wave sleep sorts and stores new knowledge so that the brain can retrieve it when you need it. Without sleep, you can learn new things, but they might not be easy to remember. This is why pulling all-nighters before tests is counterproductive for students.
- **Practicing new motor skills** - Muscle memory is actually motor planning memory. Your brain has to learn how to send a series of commands to your muscles to complete a task. Sleep is where your brain practices these sequences of actions so that you can work flawlessly when awake. Because the body is paralyzed during deep sleep, this motor practice does not result in actual actions.
- **Refining memories and forgetting unimportant details** - A few days after you learn something new, your brain will refine the memory, keeping and strengthening the important parts while forgetting extraneous details.
- **Repairing and rewiring the brain** - Neuroplasticity is a result of the work that happens during sleep. This rewiring, repairing, and interconnection happens during REM sleep.
- **Learning to navigate social situations and complex emotions** - REM sleep is how the brain learns to navigate social and emotional issues. Since more REM happens at the end of your night of sleep, people who habitually wake up to early are missing out on important social and emotional learning.
- **Creative problem-solving** - Your brain works on problems while you sleep, which is why people often come up with a brilliant solution first thing in the morning. As the brain sorts information and makes new connections, it creates solutions that you literally would not have been able to think about the night before.

This is just a brief summary of some of the more important things that sleep does for our bodies and our brains. Since sleep is such an essential part of our lives, shouldn't we want all of our patients, and everyone we love, to be getting their best possible sleep every night of their lives?

When I took Dr. Dassani's class, the pieces started to fall into place. There was an underlying cause for these symptoms, and I, as a dentist, could help them in ways that their specialists couldn't. Sleep Medicine was the missing link in the chain of specialists, and I could help them in my office, with the environment and team they already knew and loved.

Implementation on Target!

After this chapter, you'll need to do the following to get on target for your sleep dentistry practice:

- Learn the stages of sleep, and what they do for the body, by heart. You should be able to explain these to your team and patients without notes. Knowing your material makes you more persuasive.
- Learn the hormone changes with sleep.
- Be able to explain to parents, clearly and concisely, why lack of sleep impacts their children's sports and academics.
- If you're a script person, now's the time to start writing your scripts. However, I prefer to know the material inside and out, so that the patient and I can have a conversation, not a lecture.

2: Sleep Breathing: Structural Issues in Children and Adults

In this chapter you will find:

- Descriptions of OSA and UARS
- Explanations of how the tonsils and adenoids obstruct the pediatric airway
- Why tongue tie and high palates are important
- How the soft palate contributes to OSA in adults
- How the tongue and jaw affect the adult airway
- Why neck size matters

My husband had snored for years, probably as long as we'd been married. I didn't think much of it, because he'd always been that way and I could poke him when he needed to roll over. The only problem was that he got frequent sinus infections, and when those hit there was nothing anyone could do for his breathing. They took a huge toll, but his ENT had no solutions other than 'more steroids.' So we lived with it.

There are many causes of disrupted sleep, including:

- Circadian Rhythm issues
- Clock genes
- Lack of the hormone melatonin
- Poor sleep hygiene
- Difficult work schedules
- Mental illness

- Acid Reflux

In our practices, our main focus should be identifying people losing sleep due to obstructive sleep apnea (OSA). OSA occurs when structural issues restrict the airway. Because the airway is partially or totally blocked, the body can't get enough oxygen. The sleeper struggles to breathe, wakes up for a few seconds, and then slips back into sleep. These microarousals are so brief that the sleeper will not remember them in the morning. However, the work of sleep is disrupted.

We should also identify patients with upper airway resistance syndrome (UARS). UARS is often a precursor to OSA, where the patient struggles to move air through the upper airways, but can still get enough airflow to maintain oxygen levels. However, UARS patients have to work harder to breathe and the struggle results in microarousals or longer waking periods during the night. Because sleep is disrupted, the body begins a downward spiral that, if untreated, will eventually result in OSA. By identifying and treating patients with UARS, we can halt the disease process and help them avoid the weight gain, metabolic, and cardiovascular problems caused by OSA.

If we can identify the structural issues causing poor sleep, we can correct them. Dentists are the ideal providers to identify and treat OSA because we work with jaws, palates, teeth, and tongues. In most cases of OSA, these are the parts of the body that are causing or contributing to the obstruction. If a patient in your office fails a sleep screen, you'll want to conduct a physical examination to identify the source of the issues. In most cases, pediatric patients have a completely different set of structural issues than adult patients, so you'll have a different checklist for each group.

Common Obstructions in Pediatric Patients with OSA

For children with OSA, the tonsils, adenoids, tongue, and palate are often the culprits.

Tonsils and Adenoids

Tonsils and Adenoids are often severely enlarged in pediatric patients with OSA or UARS. These obstruct the airway, especially when the child is sleeping on their back. They are such a common cause of obstruction that the first line of treatment for a child with OSA is often to remove them. However, mouth-breathing can also cause the tonsils and adenoids to swell, so it's important to ensure that there isn't a more basic cause to the breathing issues.

T&A DIAGRAM FOR SURGERY

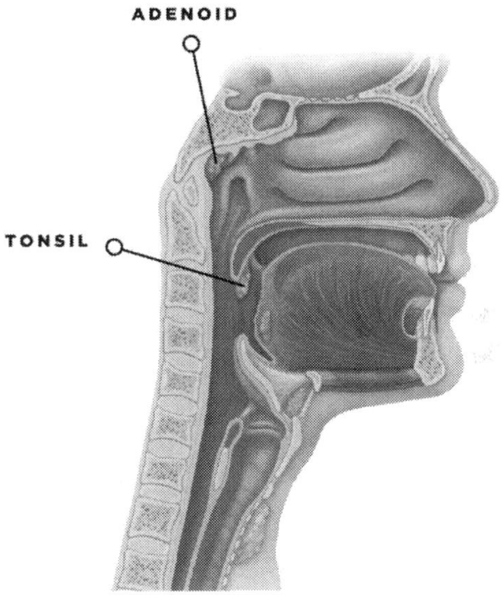

Tongue

The tongue is supposed to rest on the roof of the mouth during sleep. If it does not, it can fall backward and obstruct the stroke. In recent years, more and more children have been presenting with OSA due to an unrevised tongue-tie (ankyloglossia). This is because pediatricians and midwives have stopped revising ties unless there is a clear problem with growth and feeding. However, even children who don't have feeding issues in infancy can later have sleep issues due to tongue-tie and poor tongue positioning.

Palate

A high, narrow hard palate can obstruct breathing by reducing the volume of the nasal cavity. With the reduced volume, a slight cold or allergies can be enough to block off airflow and cause mouth-breathing and frequent night-waking. Often, a child with an unrevised tongue-tie will also have palate issues, as a normal tongue acts as a palate expander in the early years.

TONGUE TIE **HIGH PALATE** CUTAWAY DIAGRAM

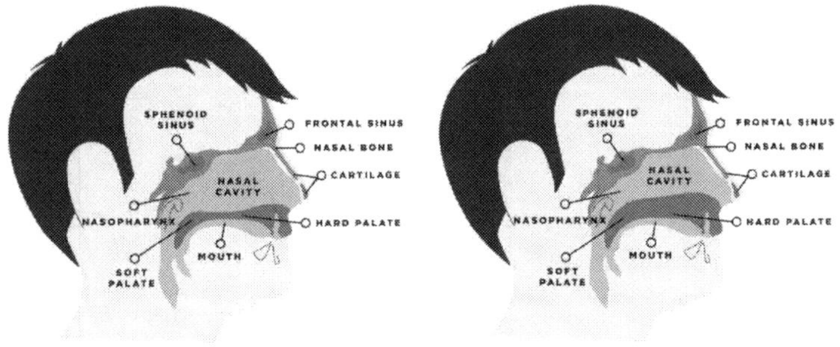

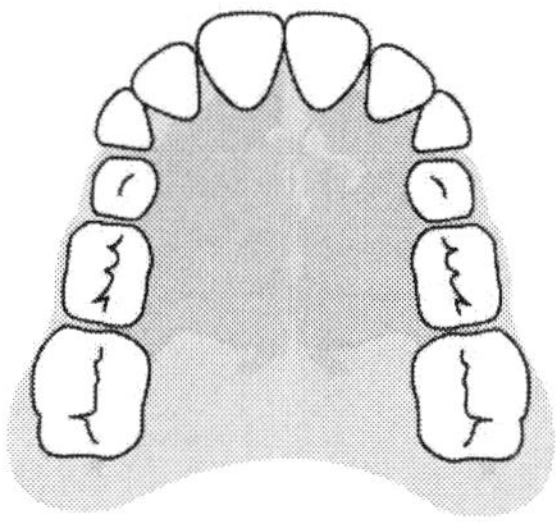

NARROW PALATE

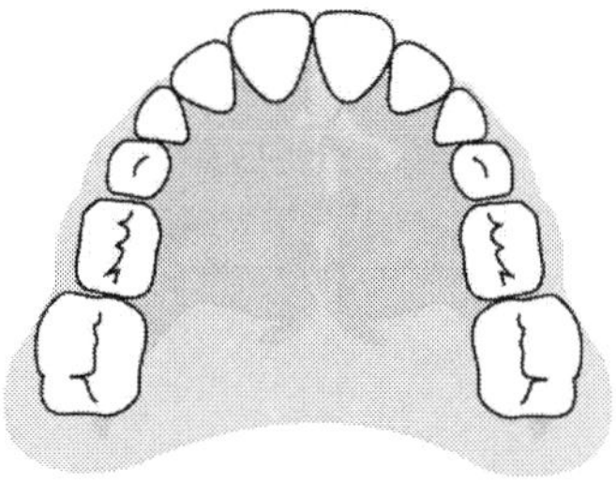

NORMAL PALATE

Common Causes of Obstruction in Adult Patients with OSA

In adults with OSA, the most common causes of obstruction are the soft palate, the tongue, the jaw, and the tissue surrounding the neck.

Soft Palate

As people age, they naturally lose muscle tone in their soft palates. During sleep, a floppy palate can fully or partially obstruct the upper airway, leading to mouth breathing or sleep apneas.

The Tongue

There are three primary ways in which the tongue can affect an adult airway during sleep:

- **Unrevised tongue tie** - We're beginning to see more and more adults whose tongue ties were not revised as infants. This can lead to the same issues with sleep breathing that it does in a child since the tongue cannot rest on the palate during sleep. Even in adults, revising a tongue tie (followed by myofunctional therapy to learn new skills), can improve sleep breathing.

- **Fatty tongue** - When people gain weight, they gain it everywhere, including on their tongues. A 2020 study from the University of Pennsylvania found that losing fat on the tongue greatly improved sleep apnea.
- **Bad habits** - If someone has fallen into the habit of mouth-breathing (perhaps from chronic sinus or allergy issues) they may have also lost the habit of proper tongue positioning during sleep. Some studies suggest that tongue exercises can alleviate this problem and improve sleep apnea.

Retrognathia

A recessed jaw impacts sleep breathing because it forces the tongue back into the throat during sleep. This narrows or blocks the airway, and can cause apneas. For patients with mild retrognathia, there are oral appliances available to position the jaw for safer sleep.

Neck Size

When there are fatty deposits in the neck, they can compress the airway during sleep and cause apneas. Adult women whose necks are more than 16 inches around and adult men whose necks are more than 17 inches around are at high risk for OSA.

Both of our kids had had tongue ties. I'd revised them myself, and they'd also both needed maxillary expansion. I knew my husband had had teeth pulled when he got braces as a kid. I knew our kids breathed much better after I'd fixed their palates, but I'd never connected the dots. I was too stuck in thinking of tongue-tie and palate issues as a pediatric issue. After the class, I realized that not only did some of my patients need treatment for sleep breathing problems, but that my husband did too. The class saved his life and his health.

Why Doesn't Everyone with Obstructions Have Full-blown OSA?

Sometimes a patient has physical features that can contribute to sleep apnea but can pass a sleep test in a lab. This is because OSA often requires multiple failures at different points in the upper respiratory syndrome. So a patient can have UARS and struggle to breathe, but not have full-blow OSA.

On the other hand, another change such as weight gain, severe allergy issues, or even an injury can then be enough to tip someone over into sleep apnea. It's important to identify treatable physical issues early so that OSA and its complications can be prevented.

Implementation on Target!

After this chapter, you should start considering how you will incorporate sleep-disordered breathing (SDB) screens into your adult and pediatric exams. For instance:

- Will you screen all new pediatric patients for tongue-tie?
- Will you alert parents to palate issues?
- Will you check the tonsils and tongue?
- For adults, will you measure neck size?
- How will you deal with evidence of an overbite?
- What will be your response to signs of tooth-grinding?

Think about these aspects of how OSA presents and start planning how your exams will change. Later, it will be important so that you can estimate how much time sleep dentistry evaluations will add to new patient and returning patient appointments.

3: Sleep Breathing: How Bad Sleep Affects Children

In this chapter, you will learn:

- Why sleep troubles can look so different in different children
- Common signs of pediatric SDB
- Why mouth-breathing is an especially significant problem

My practice had so many kids getting diagnosed with ADHD, ODD, and other behavior issues. But looking at the parents, they didn't have a history with these disorders. It's like the kids' problem just came from nowhere. It struck me as strange. With some kids who have these diagnoses, you look at the kid, and then the parents and siblings, and you can see how this is a family trait. But with some? It seemed out of the blue, and I wondered if something else was going on.

Do you have any children in your practice who have sleep-disordered breathing (SDB)? If you see pediatric patients, you almost certainly do. SDB affects about 3% of children under 12 in the US, but most children are rarely screened for it.

One reason that parents and caregivers don't have children evaluated for sleep breathing issues is that a sleepless child does not always act like a sleepless adult. For instance, compare these two "day in a life" stories for two different children.

Linnea the Lazy

Linnea was an active toddler, but as a seven-year-old, she's just lazy. She whines about chores. She whines about walks. She whines about getting up in the morning. She has a poor appetite and only wants to eat easy carbs like crackers, chips, and fruit snacks. At home, she's always bored unless she's allowed to watch her favorite shows. She slumps on the couch with her mouth open, staring at screens.

At school, Linnea spends a lot of time with her head on her desk. She's slow to speak, slow to read, and slow to do math. She can't follow two-step instructions and frequently loses her place. Whenever she's asked a question, her reply is "I don't remember." Sometimes, she breaks down crying for no good reason. Her family is nice, and her siblings are normal kids. No one can figure out what's wrong with Linnea. "Well," her teacher says, "I guess there's one in every family."

Rex the Rowdy

Rex is a ball of constant energy and poor life choices. If there's a pool, he's the one screaming "Cannonball!" and jumping in and ruining everyone's swim. If there's a dare, he'll take it. He's in the ER so often his mother has joked they should name a bay after him. Rex runs through life at full speed, never slowing down, even when he runs into something. His mom tried to put him in sports to use up some of the energy, but Rex couldn't follow directions, aggravated his teammates, and had major meltdowns whenever he was thwarted.

At school, Rex is the kid with the desk in the corner so he won't disrupt the work of the other students. He shouts out answers as soon as a question is asked, and is usually wrong. He never completes work, he won't sit still, and he's constantly acting out and getting out of his seat. His teacher wishes she could recommend an ADHD evaluation at the next parent-teacher conference because she just can't take his behavior anymore.

Which one of these children has OSA? The answer could be "Both of them!" When a child is out of sync and not getting good sleep, other variables like the family lifestyle, the child's personality, and comorbid conditions all play a role in how they behave and what issues they have.

Spotting SDB in Kids

After the seminar, I saw the pattern. These kids were kids who weren't sleeping, and who had other issues with breathing. The first parents I approached about sleep medicine were the ones who had these kids because I wanted to help the kids who were suffering most first.

Red flags for a sleep-deprived child include:

- **A habitual mouth breather** - Children breathe through their mouths when their noses and sinuses are obstructed.
- **Slack-jawed posture** - When a child is slack-jawed it can signify poor oral muscle control or poor habits, and both of these can interfere with sleep breathing.
- **Whiny with low energy levels** - This is a sign of a child who isn't getting enough sleep or who isn't breathing well enough to have energy.
- **Dampened emotions, uninterested in everything -** An exhausted child is too tired to be happy, interested, or even angry.
- **Bed-wetting** - Frequent microarousals cause the bladder to lose control. Often the problem with bedwetters is not that they sleep too deeply, but they never sleep deeply enough to concentrate urine in their sleep.
- **Poor school performance** - If a child isn't sleeping, it can be difficult for them to master new material or recall familiar material quickly.
- **Hyperactivity** - Some sleep-deprived kids are hyperactive. They seek constant stimulus to stay awake and alert, just like an adult might shake themselves, bounce up and down, or

splash cold water on their face. However, since kids are immature this stimulation takes the form of running, bouncing, talking, and acting out inappropriately.

- **Poor emotional control, including meltdowns** - Emotional control takes focus, especially for young kids. A sleep-deprived child is on an emotional rollercoaster.
- **Difficulty navigating peer relationships** - A sleep-deprived child isn't learning the skills to interact with peers and isn't able to properly process social interactions.
- **Clumsiness and poor ability to learn new gross motor skills** - Motor learning requires adequate sleep. A sleep-deprived kid will often lag behind peers in gross motor skills.
- **Restless sleep with lots of tossing and turning** - Kids with sleep issues often move a lot in their sleep, get twisted in their sheets, and fling their bodies around all night.
- **Sensory seeking or sensory avoidant behaviors** - Some kids react to exhaustion by seeking pressure, spinning, or seeking out interesting textures and sounds. Others shut down and demand silence, familiarity, and dim rooms. However, in both cases, the behavior is rooted in not being able to focus or control their feelings.
- **Snoring** - While snoring isn't always a sign of disordered breathing in a child, it can be an important indicator.
- **Dark circles under the eyes** - We also call these "allergy eyes" or "raccoon eyes." When a kid has these dark circles, it means something is interrupting their sleep.
- **Anxiety** - Sleepless kids are anxious. They know they are missing things, forgetting things, and being asked to do things they can't do, and they don't know WHY they can't act like other kids.
- **Space cadet** - Focus and short-term memory suffer when a kid doesn't sleep. So they get tagged as a space cadet who can't keep things in their brain. They lose their place in tasks easily, and can't remember what comes next.

- **Morning headaches** - Kids with breathing issues often wake dry-mouthed and with a headache.
- **Always catching respiratory bugs** - Kids with sleep breathing issues often breathe through their mouths at night. Without the nose to humidify, clean, and warm the air, they're sending too-dry, too cold, germ-laden air into their lungs. They irritate their throat and lungs and leave themselves more vulnerable to coughs and colds.

When a parent comes into your office, and you either see some of these signs in a child or they're listed on the assessment, it's time to talk to the family about sleep-disordered breathing. Often these parents have had no idea what is wrong with their child, or that there could be a common thread connecting them. Sometimes the poor child has been subjected to endless discipline in an attempt to change behaviors that they have no control over. When you identify a child with sleep-disordered breathing, you change lives.

Is Mouth-Breathing Really That Bad?

"Mouth-breather" is an insult flung in political arguments, but why is it so bad when a kid can't use her nose to breathe? They're still breathing, right? To understand just how damaging mouth-breathing can be to a child's development, it helps to learn about how it develops, why it continues, and what it does to the airways, and ultimately, to brain and body health.

How Mouth Breathing Starts

Mouth breathing usually begins when the nose and sinus cavities are blocked. The child can't get air through their nose, so they shift to their mouth. When the problem is a virus, mouth breathing is usually short-lived, and parents can take steps like steaming bathrooms or medications to open up the nose. When the mouth-breathing is the result of a longer-term problem like severe allergies or a high, narrow palate that obstructs the nasal cavity, bigger problems result.

What Happens Next

If the mouth-breathing results from a chronic condition, the child will form a habit of mouth breathing. This causes several different problems with the airway.

The nose and sinuses are essential for warming and humidifying the air that you breathe. The nose also removes particles like dust, mold, pollen, bacteria, and viruses from the air. And, of course, it allows us to smell and enhances our sense of taste.

When a child breathes through her mouth, the air enters the airway "untreated." The air irritates the tonsils, adenoids, and throat, causing inflammation, swelling, and pain. It enters the lower airway untreated and results in more irritation and inflammation.

- Mouth-breathing kids are more at risk for bronchitis, reactive airways, and asthma because their noses can't do their job. They're also more at risk for enlarged tonsils and adenoids.
- Mouth breathing positions the tongue low in the mouth instead of at the roof of the mouth. This prevents the palate from expanding properly as the child grows and also causes the tongue to block the airway during sleep, interfering with sleep breathing.
- Mouth breathing makes singing and talking more difficult. Try it. You end up gasping for breath repeatedly.
- Mouth breathing can cause a child to swallow air, and lead to GI pain.
- Mouth breathing even interferes with eating and nutrition. Kids who breathe through their mouths are often chokers. They have trouble chewing and swallowing food and drink because they can't eat and breathe at the same time. Plus, without the nose, food is just less palatable. These kids will crave super-sweet and super-salty food because that's what they can *taste.*

It all adds up to a kid who can't breathe, sleep, or eat well. And so these kids get sick more, they're always tired, they struggle with behavior and schoolwork. The longer the mouth-breathing continues, the more they miss out on and the farther they fall behind. And when mouth breathing is a habit, it takes time and effort to start nose-breathing again, even after any underlying issues are corrected. When you see a mouth-breather in your practice, it's a sign that they need your help.

The first patient we treated was a revelation. She had an unrevised tongue tie and needed her palate expanded, and the results were incredible. As she moved away from mouthbreathing and her nasal cavity expanded, her personality changed. Her parents were amazed because, inside this rage-filled, oppositional child, a sweet-tempered little girl was struggling to breathe and to rest. Now, I make sure to emphasize to parents – "Kids who don't act well probably don't feel well."

Implementation on Target!

After this chapter, do the following to help you get ready for implementation:

- Start developing or collecting educational materials for the parents of your patients. You'll want diagrams and hand-outs to explain why their child's symptoms are problematic. Virtual or physical 3D models are especially helpful for explaining the role of the palate and tongue in breathing.
- Start screening for mouth breathing. One quick question to parents, or simply watching the child breathe, can clue you and your team into bigger problems.
- Ask about school, behavioral problems, and parent worries. Many parents go into the dentist thinking "this is about teeth," so if you ask, "do you have any questions or concerns," they will only respond based on the teeth. Change how you talk to parents so that you can draw out important information.

4: Sleep Breathing: How Bad Sleep Affects Adults

If you identify sleep-disordered breathing in a child, they're likely to get treated quickly. Parents want their kids to feel better and succeed. Adults, on the other hand, will often let UARS or OSA go untreated for a long time. They're busy, the case isn't urgent, sleep studies are hard, they'll get around to it later.

When you're dealing with adult patients, it's important that they understand that untreated sleep breathing problems are very dangerous. It's not just long-term issues like diabetes or cardiovascular disease. Sleep apnea is closely linked to fatal auto accidents. Not sleeping puts you at risk of falling asleep at the wheel.

My practice had gotten busy. My life had gotten busy. I'd come home from the practice, run kids to activities and help with homework, and collapse into bed. I was working so hard to be an engaged provider for my patients, a cheerful manager for my team, and a great mom to my kids. Of course, I was exhausted and run down and running on coffee. That was normal, right?

OSA and UARS are easier to diagnose in adults than in children, simply because the symptoms tend to vary less in adults.

Mike's Story

Mike was in his 50s when he came to our practice. He'd gained weight in middle age and had just been diagnosed with high blood pressure and pre-diabetes. He was concerned because he'd been grinding his teeth, and because his wife complained about, "snores that shook the window panes." Mike worked in a factory, and recently he'd been falling asleep on his drive home from work and spacing out during the day. Mike expected to leave with a mouth guard for teeth-grinding, but instead, we sent him to a sleep lab. He had a clear-cut case of OSA. Getting treatment immediately improved his daytime sleepiness, and within a few months he was no longer pre-diabetic and his blood pressure was under control.

Gina's Story

Gina was tired all the time, but she was also a very busy person. She worked out, she had an active job, and she had two small children at home. She was slim and trim, but she just felt unhealthy. Every time she got a cold, it lingered, sometimes for weeks. She slept 8 hours every night, but she tossed and turned and her husband complained that she snored a little, every now and then. She had dark circles under her eyes that makeup couldn't hide. But when she talked to her physician about her issues, he couldn't find any evidence of an underlying problem. "It's just your time of life," he explained. "You're busy, you've got small kids, you're over 30 now. This is just what happens." By the time Gina came to us about TMJ issues, she'd given up on getting her energy back. Maybe she just was slower and less energetic than her friends and would have to learn to live with it.

OSA is Easy, UARS is Often Overlooked

Mike is a textbook OSA case. He'll have no trouble getting treatment once he gets screened and you convince him that he needs help. Gina is a harder case. She's suffering from UARS, not full-blown OSA. This means that she's struggling to breathe at night, but she still gets enough oxygen at all times. The problem is that for someone with UARS, the struggle to keep breathing triggers microarousals and they toss, turn, and change position. Remember, to do the work of sleep, the body needs to *STAY* asleep. Gina's microarousals mean that her body and brain can't heal the way they should. Her hormones are out of whack because she's not sleeping deeply enough for long enough. Right now, she is healthy, but if she can't get help the damage will pile up. She'll end up with cardiovascular disease, T2 Diabetes, obesity, and full-blown OSA because she is not sleeping.

In some ways, a UARS patient will receive a GREATER benefit from treatment than an OSA patient will because if you can catch sleep breathing issues early, you can prevent chronic diseases like diabetes.

So, the sleep course was eye-opening. I recognized myself in the symptoms and realized that I'd been assuming OSA was for old, slow, overweight people, not young, trim, active moms in their 30s! I was my own first sleep patient because I wanted my energy back. I wasn't 100% sold on making sleep dentistry a major focus of my practice, but I started treating family and friends. At that point, it wasn't a business decision. I felt better and I wanted the people I loved to feel better too.

Common Signs of SDB in Adults

The most common signs of UARS or OSA in adults include:

- **Snoring** - Either because a partner complained or because they wake themselves up.
- **Gasping, choking, and stop-breathing episodes** - (Usually reported by a partner.)
- **Falling asleep at the wheel, for short periods** - This is very dangerous and always a medical emergency because car accidents can be deadly.
- **Nodding off at work** - These microsleeps can affect careers, as the sleeper may not appear to be asleep and may agree to assignments while asleep.
- **Craving salty and sweet food and being unable to eat healthy foods** - This is a result of the hormone changes from sleep deprivation. The brain craves fast, satisfying hits to keep it awake.

- **Lack of willpower or ability to make changes** - An unrested brain gets stuck in its ways and it's harder to make changes, learn new things, or develop new habits.
- **Weight gain, and the inability to lose weight even when dieting and exercising** - However, if a person has UARS, they may NOT be overweight yet.
- **High blood pressure**
- **Type 2 diabetes or prediabetes**
- **Aching joints and muscles**
- **Waking frequently at night**
- **High, narrow palate**
- **Overbite**
- **Insomnia, inability to stay asleep**
- **Anxiety about falling asleep**
- **Treatment-resistant depression or anxiety**
- **Drug or alcohol addiction. This is often self-medication for sleep issues**
- **Trouble learning more material** - This symptom often shows up when someone goes back to school.
- **Exhaustion, needing frequent rests during everyday tasks**
- **Brain fog**
- **Large neck size**
- **Dry mouth in the morning**
- **Waking with a headache**
- **Inability to get out of bed, even after 8 hours of "sleep"**
- **Inattention**
- **Irritability**

One of the best ways to screen an adult patient for SDB, besides questionnaires, is to just spend a few moments talking to them about their lives. Ask for details. How often do they feel exhausted? What tasks exhaust them? What did they use to be able to do, that they can't anymore? Fleshing out these little details gives a clearer picture of the problem, and gives you a way to explain the concrete benefits of getting their sleep issues treated.

It was a conversation with my mom that hammered it home. I'd treated her OSA, and she felt great. She told me, flat out, "You have to offer this to all your patients. There's a real need. Stop letting fear hold you back. Why should our family be the only ones who benefit from your new knowledge?" She was right, of course. Once I committed to implementing sleep dentistry, I was never short of sleep patients.

Implementation on Target!

After this chapter you should:

- Create a plan for how you'll screen for SDB. Ensure that everyone, not just, "Stereotypical OSA patients" will get screened.
- Start collecting or creating educational materials including 3D digital or physical models of the upper airway, handouts about OSA and UARS, and images to explain the conditions to your patients.
- Identify a few patients who may benefit from being "guinea pigs" for sleep medicine.
- Consider how long an annual checkup that includes both oral cancer screen and sleep screening will need to be.

5: Team First: Using Education to Build Your Office Sleep Squad

In this chapter you will learn:

- How to approach your team about sleep dentistry
- How different parts of the team will be involved in implementation, and how to involve them in the planning process
- How team member personality types affect implementation goals

If you've ever read a business book, you're familiar with this common scenario:

The CEO of a company has a great idea. She's going to take the company in a new direction and reach a new market. It will be great! But, when it comes time to actually implement her idea, the CEO falls flat. It seems like her team is working against her. Everyone has dug in. They're grumbling in the break rooms. No one is willing to buy into her great idea and do the work to make it happen.

At this point, whichever consultant is writing the book usually steps in to explain how to communicate to different types of personalities, how to engage everyone, and how to get the company on board with this new idea.

I came back from the sleep seminar pumped up and ready to implement. Sleep dentistry was a great way to serve my patients and expand the practice. I was ready to go! And then I hit a wall. My team was furious with me. They thought I was hopping on a fad and that we were going to mess up all our processes for no good reason. I had been so excited about the medicine behind sleep dentistry that I forgot I needed ***people*** *to implement it, not just knowledge.*

I want you to be able to skip the step where everything fails and you're angry, and go straight to a team that's excited about sleep dentistry and all-in on implementation. How do you do that? By educating them about what a difference they can make.

If you haven't attended a sleep seminar yet, stop right now. You'll have the best luck on implementation if you have some of your team attend with you. Your hygienists, assistants, and office staff will all take different things away from a seminar, and chances are that they'll have implementation ideas that never occurred to you. So, if you haven't attended yet, plan on attending as a practice.

For the rest of you, it's important to be excited about sleep dentistry, but your excitement alone won't be enough to get your team on board. You need to get them excited too.

Phase 1: You Just Finished Your Seminar and You Are Totally Pumped

This is a great place to be. You've learned about sleep apnea and sleep dentistry, you've gotten to spend time with other excited people, and you have lots of plans and notes and dreams. So what next?

The first step is to pass this enthusiasm on to your staff. That means a big team meeting, maybe an in-service day, right? Not so fast. If you go straight to a meeting, this becomes a top-down implementation. It might work, but it will take a lot of constant mental effort on your part. Instead, aim for a "bubble up from the bottom" implementation. Get your team excited first so that they'll be eager to take on new responsibilities and rearrange their routines.

To do this:

- Talk to people one on one. If your front desk person asks how the seminar went, tell her! Share something cool you learned about sleep and learning, or about sleep and whole-body health. Do this with other team members too. Even mention it to patients where your hygienists and assistants can listen.
- After you've had a chance to share your enthusiasm with most of the team one-on-one, bring it to a short morning meeting. "I learned about this, I think it could help us, our practice, and our patients, does anyone else want to learn more?"
- Take volunteers and have them learn more about sleep medicine. My book *Airway is Life* is a great place to start, since it's a quick read and written for general audiences. If they're interested, you may find it worthwhile to have them complete an online sleep seminar for CE credit. They won't get the same things out of it that you did, but they'll have different insights based on their own roles in the practice.
- Once you have some of the team on board, it's time to educate the rest of the team. Block out a morning or afternoon, and teach them about sleep! Start with why lack of sleep harms adults and kids, and then go right to "How we, as a dental practice, can help."

So, I had to take a few steps back. I realized I had to sell everyone on sleep dentistry, and that meant selling everyone on the science of sleep. My team is like most busy American women. They have too much to do, not enough time to do it, and routinely short themselves on sleep and then hit the coffee hard all day long. So, instead of starting right in on sleep dentistry and how to implement it, we started with "why you need sleep and how your mind and body break down when you're not getting enough." And, of course, they all saw themselves in that, because of their busy lifestyles.

Phase 2: Breaking Down the Steps and Timeline

After the team understands why OSA is important and what your practice can do to improve health and save lives, it's time for each department to think about how their jobs will change, and how long it will take to implement those changes. You'll want to meet with each department individually, as this is a lot to think about. And if people need time to get back to you with a schedule, book a second meeting as well.

You delegate to your department heads because they know their jobs and you trust them. Give them a chance to be trustworthy in implementing sleep dentistry, too!

Your Job

There are a few pieces of the implementation puzzle that only you can do. You'll need to give yourself deadlines for each of these tasks. If it helps, make another member of the team your accountability partner to help you stay on track. I know you're busy with your current routines, but to get the benefits of sleep dentistry you first must make time for the set-up process.

- **Reaching out to specialists and other providers -** A member of your team can research the lists of potential partners and provide contact info, but in the end, you're going to have to be the person to make contact. You're the provider, you have training and knowledge, you can't outsource this person-to-person communication to a member of the office team. Keep in mind that it may take 1-3 "touches" to make contact with your specialists and referring physicians. Try to reach them by calling, email, *and* a physical letter. This part takes patience and can be stressful and boring. Do it anyway. It's essential for the success of your sleep dentistry program.
- **Practicing your physical OSA exams for adults and pediatric patients -** This takes practice. You'll need a few volunteers so that you can hone your routine and get faster. See if friends, family, and team members are willing to be your first patients.

After you've practiced, you'll have a better idea about how long a sleep exam takes you and how your appointment blocking will need to change to incorporate Sleep Dentistry.

- **Make contact with vendors, demo various oral appliances and technologies, and choose a few favorites** - There are many OSA appliances on the market, and each one has a different set of strengths and weaknesses. Demo them, get to see them in person, and develop opinions. Pick a favorite, but make sure you're also educated about all your options so that you can meet the needs of each patient.

Scheduling

A sleep program will add a few minutes to every standard appointment, as we screen for and discuss sleep issues. In addition, if a patient reports issues during a screen, it may result in a longer-than-usual exam. During the ramp-up phase, everyone's appointment is likely to be longer. After that, it will only be new patients and patients with new symptoms.

- Can we immediately increase the length of New Patient appointments to incorporate sleep medicine? If not, when can we do that?
- Is there a way to make every returning patient's next check-up include sleep medicine for one cycle of appointments? (So that, starting 6 months from today and until 12 months from today, each recare appointment is longer, but they go back to normal after that?)
- Do we have enough elasticity in the schedule to incorporate sleep dentistry? If not, how do we need to change our blocking?
- How quickly can we adjust our blocks to allow space for sleep dentistry

Front Desk

The front desk will need to add sleep screening checklists to the material that each patient gets on check-in. These should be completed at every visit so that the office can track changes over time and catch problems in the early stages. Ask:

- Who will create these forms?
- How long will that take?
- How will they be added to the patient packets?
- Is there a way to have patients complete them online before they arrive?
- Who will we contact to implement that?
- How long will it take?

Hygiene Team

The hygiene team's role in adding sleep dentistry is very organic. During their part of appointments, team members should look to see if they spot any hints of potential OSA, and alert you to any findings, just as they already do with other dental and health issues.

- Can you add measures such as neck circumference to your initial exam?
- Which signs of OSA (bruxism, palate issues, etc.) can you identify during your time with the patient?
- How will you flag issues for the doctor to signal that the patient needs extra time and attention due to sleep issues?
- What educational materials such as posters or brochures and flyers can you put in your bay to make patients more aware of OSA?
- Are you comfortable talking about OSA, or do you need scripts?
- How quickly can you adjust your routine to include OSA screening and conversation?

Billing Team

The billing team also has an important role in implementation. We implement sleep dentistry for the good of patients and communities, but we also implement it for the good of our practices. It's important to get paid for the important new services that you and your team are offering. If you have a strong billing team, this is their time to shine. Let them own the process and do their own problem-solving. After all, they're more experienced with billing than you are. Ask:

- How familiar are you with medical billing? Which procedures are you already familiar with?
- When will you be available to attend a session on medical billing for sleep dentistry?
- Which medical insurers are most common in our area? How do we contract with them?
- What documentation will you need for our sleep medicine program?
- How will we allow patients to finance treatments that insurance will not cover?
- Which procedures will be billed as medical and which will be billed as dental?

Social Media and Marketing Teams

I am not going to go in-depth into marketing in this book. I've found that once you have good relationships with patients and providers, word of mouth is the best marketing possible for your sleep program. However, we all have blogs and Facebook and Instagram, and we all plan posts. So while you don't need a marketing blitz, give your team a schedule for when they can expect your sleep dentistry program to ramp up and make sure that mentions of OSA and sleep dentistry make it into your social media presence.

Once they had a basic understanding of sleep, and OSA and UARS, a few of my team wanted to be screened. What hammered it home was that, over time, untreated OSA can lead to weight gain, high blood pressure, and diabetes. No one wanted to deal with that. So I did a screening and exam on the team members who had volunteered as "guinea pigs." My team was starting to get engaged with the process.

A Quick Note on Office Personalities and Adding Sleep Dentistry

In his book *Surrounded by Idiots,* international communication expert Thomas Erikson discusses why different personality types resist workplace change – and how you can help them adjust and contribute. Thomas uses a traditional 4-quadrant personality map.

Reds, or the Cholorics, are the typical type A personality. They like to lead, get ahead, and win. They like information to be short, focused, and to the point. They enjoy change, especially if it can be cast as "progress."

Yellows, or Sanguines, are natural cheerleaders. They love people and communicating, and excitement. They're not great on details or follow-through, but they're important for making others feel social and happy. They also love change, as long as there aren't too many fussy little bits to pay attention to.

Greens, or Phlegmatics, are humanitarians and relationship people, but they also like predictability. They change slowly, need clear goals, and need to understand the "why" of what is happening to feel comfortable.

And finally, Blues, or Melancholics, are extremely detail-oriented. They want to get everything right but often won't point out your mistakes unless you ask.

Most people are a mix of 2 or 3 colors, but when change happens one color comes to the fore in sharp relief. Take a few minutes and think about your team. Can you see who fits under which color without too much effort?

So what does this have to do with communicating to your team about sleep medicine?

Because Dentistry is a helping profession, you probably have many Yellows and Greens on your team. Yellows are especially concentrated at front desks and as social media marketers. They're enthusiastic. Talk to them about helping people, and they're off. They'll be your sleep medicine evangelists, and they'll be great in that role.

You'll probably find that many of your hygienists are green. They are affable, like helping people, and like the predictability of their days. They're not in dentistry to get ahead and take out the competition. They're here because they love the patients and the work. To get your greens on board, explain the reasons for sleep medicine. They're the ones who will be interested in the medical reasons to treat OSA and the fact that screening and treatment makes lives better. By showing them how this is an extension of the work you're already doing, you'll get them on board. Just make sure you have some scripts and checklists to help them through the transition.

I hope, very much, that your scheduling and billing teams have a decent proportion of blues. These are, perhaps, the hardest changes to make to add sleep dentistry and you'll need someone who can be detail-oriented, plan carefully, and prepare for all contingencies. Blues love being right, so try not to micromanage here. Tell them what you need, and ask THEM the best way to get from here to there.

Finally, Reds. If you're a dentist who loves growing and stomping out the competition, you might be a red. But Reds are generally drawn to tournament professions, not ones that demand careful, steady commitment day after day. If part of the reason you're adding sleep dentistry is that you want to spend more time with your family and to help people, you're probably also mostly green. HOWEVER, the practice does need a strong leader to implement the program.

So, try to channel a little bit of that red energy right now, and lead your team towards a future with a thriving sleep dentistry program.

Phase 3: Go Time!

You've laid the groundwork and gotten your team excited and invested in the process. You've let everyone in the office know that they have a job to do to make this a success. Everyone is busy learning about OSA and optimizing their own roles for the new program.

Finally, you're ready to dive in and get started with the act of implementation. By taking time to plan first, you've set yourself, your team, and your patients up for success.

One of the team wanted a sleep study after her screening. She had UARS. Her lifestyle is more suited to an appliance than a PAP machine, so I made her one. Within two weeks, she was a sleep evangelist. My team could see the difference in her, and I could see how it clicked with them. They realized we were doing real medicine and meeting a real need, and resistance to implementation evaporated.

Implementation on Target!

After this chapter, you should:

- Have found the "sleep evangelists" on your team and talked to them about your hopes and goals for this program
- Planned a team meeting to divide up timelines and responsibilities
- After the meeting, you should have a clear schedule for implementation. Put this somewhere public and obvious, like the break room.
- Be prepared to check in with your various groups, see how the process is going, and find out if they've encountered any roadblocks.

Part 2: Implementing Adult Sleep Dentistry

You may be wondering why I've chosen to break out adult sleep dentistry implementation from pediatric implementation. There are several ways in which adult sleep dentistry differs from pediatric sleep dentistry:

- You're talking to, and educating, the patient and their partner, not the parents.
- You'll work with a slightly different set of physicians and specialists.
- The solutions for SDB in an adult are often different than the solutions for a child.
- Not all sleep dentistry practices treat pediatric patients.

However, if you're currently only planning to practice pediatric sleep dentistry, I'd still suggest you read this chapter, for two important reasons. First of all, we're increasingly seeing something more similar to adult SDB in older teens, so even a pediatric dental practice could benefit. On the other hand, if you run a family dental practice, you may find that the parents of your pediatric sleep dentistry patients may also come to you for help and support.

Now that you understand the basics of sleep science and getting your team on board, you're ready to fully implement adult sleep dentistry. Let's get to work!

6: Where Will My Patients Come From?

In this chapter you'll learn:

- Which of your adult patients need sleep medicine
- Why specialists need your special expertise
- How you can get all the sleep patients you need with minimal marketing

One of the most common questions my students ask is about finding patients. Where will all of the sleep dentistry patients come from? Often, they're looking for a specific marketing plan. They want to know how much to spend on advertising, how much on social media, where to place promotions, and how long to run them for.

I have disappointing news for all of your marketing consultants and teams. I find that I don't need to advertise at all. Add a sleep dentistry services page to your website, maybe occasionally mention it in a social post, and you're good. How can this be?

Because sleep medicine is such a high-demand specialty that your patients will come to you. Once you start screening your existing patients and working with providers, you will have a constant stream of patients looking for help, and you'll be there to provide it to them!

My first sleep patients were family. I'd come back from the seminar weighted down by the knowledge that my parents, aunts and uncles, and cousins needed my help, and fast. So, I got them in first, and then did a soft launch, just screening a few high-risk patients. I couldn't believe how quickly it snowballed.

Younger Adults Need Medical Care

25% of American adults have no primary care provider, and 40% of adults in their 20s and 30s don't have a relationship with a physician. These are the people who see a Doc-in-a-Box for the occasional sinus infection, get their shots at the pharmacy, or maybe have an onsite clinic at work. They don't go in for check-ups and no one is screening them for sleep issues.

Even among Americans who have good insurance and a primary care provider, more than half do not see their doctor at least once a year. Younger, healthier people are more likely to skip the doctor.

Meanwhile, some people don't see doctors but ARE careful about their teeth and who see you every six months, like clockwork. Not only that, but people choose you as their dentist because they like you and trust you. Dental appointments can be scary and uncomfortable, if they're coming in it's because they know you care about them and their health.

There's a good chance your patients under 40, in particular, are not receiving regular medical care, except in your office. This means that if they have UARS or OSA, no one is catching it. Years of bad sleep pile up and create lasting damage to the body.

If you can give that young woman with UARS an appliance now, her condition may not advance to OSA. She'll dodge the weight gain, the cardiovascular issues, the emotional issues, and the memory issues associated with poor sleep. You could prevent a fatal car crash. Not only that, but she'll have years to advance in her career that she wouldn't have had if she'd struggled with poor sleep for another decade or two.

So, what is the first step to getting patients for your sleep dentistry practice? ***Screening ALL your existing patients.***

People Don't Love the PAP Machine

One of the biggest barriers to care for people with UARS or OSA is that many people cannot tolerate the PAP machines. In studies, researchers commonly find that between 30-80% of people with OSA cannot hit the bare minimum for compliance, even when they know their use is being watched and recorded. (Usually, you'd expect people to do better if they know they're getting a "grade" for success, so these numbers suggest that in real life, compliance is even worse.)

This is especially terrible because "compliance" is defined as using the PAP for at least 4 hours a night on 70% of nights. If we assume most people need 7-8 hours of sleep uninterrupted by microarousals, then even PAP users aren't getting enough rest. Plus, 30% of the time they may not even be getting 4 hours in!

People with asthma, allergies, sinus issues, and dry eyes have a difficult time complying with PAP therapy. The machines also disturb people who need quiet to sleep, and they're not workable for people who share the bed with pets, who change position while sleeping, or who have to get up frequently to care for small children.

Problems with compliance may be one reason why PAP machines seem to slow the progression of SDB-related issues, but not entirely stop them. ***A treatment is only a treatment if the patient can actually comply with it.***

Meanwhile, OAT for SDB has a higher compliance rate, especially as time goes on. People who have appliances tend to make them part of their routine and pop them in before bed at night. They leave them in all night and take them out in the morning. When a patient has an oral appliance for their sleep apnea, they comply with treatment.

When used perfectly, PAP machines often outperform oral appliances, which makes sense. The machine literally forces air into the airways. However, a machine that sits unused is not keeping the airway open or getting oxygen to the brain. For many of your patients, the revelation that an oral appliance similar to the retainer they wore as a kid can improve their breathing will seem almost miraculous. Simply educating existing patients with OSA diagnoses about alternative treatments can help your sleep dentistry practice grow.

I couldn't believe how many of my regular patients had daytime sleepiness, morning headaches, and were in the early stages of high blood pressure and type 2 diabetes. Most had never had a sleep screen at a doctor's appointment. They said their doctors just told them to try and lose weight and eat better, but never brought up the idea of sleep apnea as an underlying cause.

Specialists Need Your Help

The other main source of adult sleep dentistry patients for your practice is referrals from primary care providers and specialists. It's not just your patients who have problems complying with PAP therapy. This is a universal problem. General Practitioners, Pulmonologists, Cardiologists, Endocrinologists, and ENTs all have patients who have OSA but who can't tolerate the PAP machines. Often, these specialists know that oral appliance therapy exists, but are unsure who offers it. They may counsel patients to "ask your dentist at your next appointment," without having the name of a specific dentist in mind.

Once you reach out to these specialists in your community, you'll have plenty of patients. Sleep dentistry is an area where the most effective marketing is based on personal relationships and recommendations. People are suffering, they need solutions, and you are there to help them. You can market more if you enjoy marketing, but it's not a necessary part of the implementation process.

Getting Sleep Patients the Easy Way

With these facts in mind, there are several steps you cannot skip if you want to have a good stream of sleep dentistry patients.

1. **Get the team on board** - I know I had a whole chapter devoted to this earlier, but this is the most important step. If your team is unenthusiastic about or hostile to the idea of sleep dentistry, all your attempts at getting sleep patients will fail. You must educate, train and persuade your team that sleep dentistry is good for their careers, the practice, and the patients.
2. **Collect or produce educational materials** - Aim for several levels from a basic overview to a few higher-level materials to share with specialists and with patients who get very excited about sleep medicine. Have these ready so that when people ask for more information, you're prepared. If you have to get back to them later, they won't get back to you.
3. **Learn the science by heart** - Study the science behind sleep until you can talk about it naturally and without stress. Good teachers know their material, and the way you'll get sleep medicine cases is by educating patients and doctors.
4. **Build good relationships with specialists** - We'll go into more detail on this later, but you must build these relationships before you start your first sleep case. What good is telling someone they have SDB if you can't refer them to the proper specialists for diagnosis?
5. **Talk to patients, friends, family, and community members** - You've learned exciting things and you're about to start doing important work. Tell people. Educate the people around you about sleep and health, and they'll spread the word for you.

"I'm Really Not Comfortable Not Marketing. What Can I Do?"

If you can't let go and let patients come to you without marketing, I'd suggest the following easy ways to get the word out about your new sleep dentistry program:

- **Your website** - When you're ready to launch, add a services page.

- **Your social media** - Share sleep facts, and info about your new program, as part of your social media routine.
- **A launch party** - When you introduce sleep dentistry, celebrate it! This has a dual purpose – it builds excitement for your team ***and*** gets information out to your patients and possibly community news sources.
- **Lectures at your library or other community groups** - Did you know that many community groups, like Kiwanis, are always in search of speakers for their luncheons? And libraries often offer health and wellness programming. Even your local 4-H or agricultural extension offices may be interested in offering sleep programming if you offer to give talks. This is a national health crisis, and when you get the word out to your community, you get patients.

You'll notice that most of these are variations on word-of-mouth marketing or authority marketing. That's because, for a targeted service like this one, just educating people and spreading the word that you can help will bring in new patients.

What Sort of Materials Should I Have to Talk to People About Sleep Dentistry?

Since you'll be reaching out to specialists, team members, and the general public, you'll need to have a toolset of props, pictures, and handouts to explain sleep apnea.

Some useful materials include:

- **A cutaway model of the upper airway** - These are available at reasonable prices online. While images are helpful, sometimes being able to touch the various parts of the airway helps your audience understand the issues more clearly.
- **A model of the mouth, teeth, and tongue, with movable tongue** - This can help you explain how the position of the tongue matters to the airway. Speech therapists use these to help children understand tongue position.

- **Handouts (single sheet or trifold)** - These should address specific questions and concerns about what causes OSA, what the effects are, and treatment options. As you practice sleep dentistry, you'll probably find that you need to expand your materials. The key is that all of these should have interesting and informative visuals, concise text, and your office's contact information.
- **Testimonials/true stories** - After you've treated your first few sleep dentistry patients, get testimonials and start using those as part of your materials. Even when people understand the science, tying it to stories of real people makes it more memorable.
- **A CPAP and an oral appliance** - People will want to see how big PAP machines are, what the masks are like, and how they sound when they're plugged in. They'll also want to see oral appliances and how they differ from a normal retainer. Touching helps some people learn and remember, so have these in your "sleep apnea toolkit."
- **A PowerPoint presentation to organize your charts, graphs, and visuals** - A PowerPoint is a great way to organize your visuals because you can click on the most relevant one for the conversation you're having. You should also store some of your favorites on your phone, so you can easily pull them up during 1-to-1 conversations about sleep dentistry.

As you continue to educate people about sleep dentistry inside and outside your practice, you'll find other tools that help you communicate to your community. When you find a need, fill it! Soon you'll have a reputation as the local sleep dentist.

I still don't market my sleep dentistry program, other than by giving educational talks at local events and organizations, and that's more about being a good citizen than actual marketing. Instead, every time I help someone new, they spread the word to their family and friends. There is a huge need for sleep dentistry. So many PAP machines sit abandoned in corners, and people are living with untreated OSA because they don't realize that an appliance is an option! I found that once you take the leap and just get started treating sleep patients, the program grows itself.

Implementation on Target!

After this chapter you should:

- Order any models you need to explain sleep science.
- Memorize the key facts of sleep science and OSA so that you can explain them without having to look at notes or mentally reach for information.
- Make a list of places you'd like to do community outreach, and contact numbers for those places.
- Put together your PowerPoint.
- Plan your launch. What date are you launching? Will you tease it first? Where? Where will you launch?

Sources for this chapter:

https://www.reuters.com/article/us-health-pcp-trends/declining-numbers-of-americans-have-a-primary-care-provider-idUSKBN1YK1Z4

https://www.sleepreviewmag.com/sleep-treatments/therapy-devices/cpap-pap-devices/top-10-practices-to-increase-cpap-compliance/

https://erj.ersjournals.com/content/50/suppl_61/PA4725

7: Reaching out to the Doctors and Specialists in Your Area

In this chapter you'll learn:

- Which specialists you should build relationships with
- How to educate specialists about oral appliance therapy (OAT)
- How to contact and speak to specialists
- Who to make your first referrals to
- How to overcome roadblocks to your referral network

It is impossible to start a successful adult sleep program on your own. To practice sleep dentistry, you'll need connections with a host of specialists. At a bare minimum, set up a mutual referral system with:

- At least one ENT practice
- At least one sleep lab
- At least one primary care physician group

In addition, it can be helpful to build strong connections with:

- An allergist
- A cardiologist
- A pulmonologist
- An SLP
- A myofunctional therapist

- An endocrinologist
- A pharmacist

How do you find these specialists, build relationships, and bring them into your Sleep Dentistry Team? In this chapter, I'll outline a process that you can use to forge these connections. You don't have to follow it step-by-step. Every community is different, you may spot some shortcuts that will work in yours. However, if you're lost and unsure of your next steps, this guide will help you build your team.

One of the hardest parts for me about this stage of implementation was outsourcing the research to other team members. I wanted to be in control and find the right specialists, but I just didn't have the time to identify partners, reach out, and build relationships, so my program was floundering. Looking back, I should have done this first, and I should have delegated it to a team member.

Finding Specialists:

Step 1: Making the Lists

So, how will you decide which physicians and specialists you'll contact about your sleep dentistry program? The first step is to find out who is working in sleep medicine in your area. Start with your family's own physicians, ENT, etc. Even if they're not a perfect fit for your program, you already know them and may find it less awkward to approach them.

If you have kids in school, think about the other parents you already know. Are any of them in the proper medical fields? If so, they might be worth approaching, especially if you already get along and have worked well together on school or sports-related projects.

For primary care physicians who can partner with you, your practice management software is a great place to start. Do you collect data on a patient's physician? Use it! See which PCPs and practices are most popular with your patients, and add them to your list.

After you've collected the easy names, it's time for research. You can delegate this task to the team member who usually handles billing and insurance. Which hospitals and physician groups are in-network for the most popular insurers in your area? What specialists or groups might help implement a sleep program? For each specialty, collect both a name and a backup, in case your first choice isn't interested in the program yet. Have your team member record all contact info – office number, phone, address, email, website.

Step 2: Focus on Developing Educational Programs

A great way to add to your list of potential specialists and to increase interest in your sleep dentistry program is to offer educational programming. Are there study groups for physicians and specialists in your area, either independently or through a hospital system? Volunteer to offer a program and provide food.

Most physicians only receive a brief introduction to sleep medicine in medical school or their residencies. Many have no idea that oral appliance therapy has been proven to be an effective treatment for UARS and mild to moderate OSA. So, get out there and educate your local medical community! Bring notepads or business cards with your office information along. Many physicians have patients who can't tolerate the CPAP but don't know how to get them help. You have a solution to their problems, you just have to let them know who you are and what you are doing.

Step 3: Making Contact

The next step is to reach out to the people on your list. Keep in mind that you may have to contact them more than once before you get a response. Start with a letter explaining what your new sleep program will entail, why you're contacting them, and how to get in touch with you to discuss options. You can also include a form for them to return if they'd like to be part of a mutual referral program.

Your letter may look something like this. Feel free to take this general format and customize it for your own practice and specialists.

February 2, 2022

Dear Dr. Jones,

I am a local dentist who is adding sleep dentistry to my practice. Sleep dentistry identifies and treats patients with Sleep Disordered Breathing in a dental practice setting through the use of appliances that correct palate issues, improve tongue positioning, and keep the airway open during sleep.

To successfully reach these patients and improve their health, I need to be able to refer them to a <insert specialty> for a sleep study and diagnosis. May I refer these patients to your office for care?

While I am adding this service to benefit my existing patients, I am also able to take referrals for non-patients who have trouble fitting PAP therapy into their lives and who would like to try a custom oral appliance as an alternative. Oral appliance therapy for Upper Airway Resistance Syndrome (UARS) and mild-to-moderate Obstructive Sleep Apnea (OSA) can be especially helpful for people who travel and camp a lot, who have asthma or allergies that make PAP use difficult, or whose partners find the PAP machine annoying.

I am passionate about getting as many people as possible help for their sleep breathing problems, and therapy is only effective if patients can comply with it. Please let me know if your office can help my patients by accepting referrals for diagnosis.

Sincerely,

<name>

After you send the letter, you need to follow up. Even if a physician is willing to partner with your sleep medicine program, they may set the letter aside, intending to respond later. About 14 days after the letters are mailed, you should follow up with a phone call. In most cases, you'll talk to the office manager, not the physician. In the call you should:

- Ask the letter was received
- Ask if the physician has any questions
- Ask if there is a specific fax, phone, or email to use when referring patients
- Offer to send another letter
- Leave your contact information

Step 4: Choose a Team Member to Work on These Relationships

Good relationships take work. It's a cliché from self-help books, but it also applies to your relationships with other specialists. If the clinical side of the practice keeps you too busy to maintain relationships with the physicians who you refer to and who refer to you, then a team member needs to step in to follow through.

One way to manage these relationships is with a simple spreadsheet or table.

Keep track of how many referrals go back and forth between your practices, what your last contact with each office was, and when you should get back in touch with them. Examples of contacts are:

- Updates on patients
- Thank you notes for referrals or for helping a patient get diagnosed
- Newsletters
- Small tokens of appreciation
- Calls
- Visits to their office by you or a team member
- Emails
- Meetings at luncheons or other professional events
- Direct mailers
- Facebook and LinkedIn connections
- Local professional groups online and in-person

The more personalized your contacts can be, the better. You want these other practitioners to remember that you exist, that you appreciate their help with your patients, and that you provide great care to their patients. Frequent contacts mean that when they have a patient who can't tolerate PAP therapy or who has underlying teeth, tongue, or palate issues, they'll think of you.

To keep up with these relationships, choose a team member who is outgoing, cheerful, and intelligent. If their current duties won't give them time to help build your referral program, it's time to change up job descriptions and redistribute workloads. Building a good 2-way referral network is essential for practicing sleep dentistry.

Step 5: Making Your First Sleep Dentistry Referrals

Once you've begun to make contact with the specialists in your areas, you can make your first sleep dentistry referrals, perhaps as part of a beta test (see Chapter 12). Eventually, you'll develop bidirectional relationships with these specialists, but for now, it's up to you to take the first step.

You've identified a patient who needs a sleep study. Who do you call? If they have a good relationship with their PCP, you can start there. Otherwise, which specialist do you plan to work with for sleep studies and to diagnose UARS and OSA?

When you make the referral, first talk to the patient. Explain that as a dentist, you can't order a sleep study or diagnose UARS/OSA (unless, according to the American Academy of Dental Sleep Medicine, you practice in Idaho, Louisiana, Maryland, Mississippi, or South Dakota, in which case you are permitted to order and interpret sleep studies.) Inform the patient that, to complete the diagnostic process, you'll be referring them to another doctor, who you trust to take good care of them.

Have your office team call in the referral and set up an appointment for your patient. It's important to complete this step before the patient leaves the office. Otherwise, they may intend to set up an appointment later, but never get around to it.

Check with the patient after their appointment to see how it went, and follow up with the doctor that you referred them to. Were they sent for a sleep study? Why or why not? If they were not sent for a sleep study, what documentation does the doctor need to order one?

Some specialists are more conservative about diagnosing sleep-disordered breathing than others. This can be a problem since waiting for UARS to progress to OSA or mild OSA to progress to severe OSA means that your patient's body will undergo irreversible damage. The earlier that we can identify and treat SDB, the more health problems we can prevent.

If you find that you are referring to a specialist who doesn't take your observations or your patients' experiences seriously, stop. Find a new specialist who is willing to diagnose UARS and mild OSA so that your patients can get help before their disease progresses to weight gain, high blood pressure, or diabetes.

Step 6: Make Sure You Follow Up

Follow up with your patient and the specialist to find out when their sleep study occurred and what the results are. If they were borderline for OSA or UARS, remember that symptoms matter. If someone is subclinical on a sleep study but falls asleep at the wheel, it's a medical emergency and their SDB is not actually subclinical.

If you need to pull together extra documentation for insurance, now is the time. The Epworth Sleepiness Scale can be a big help here. So can evidence of tooth grinding. Resubmit your evidence to the specialist, and keep pushing for a diagnosis. Your patient needs help, or they're running the risk of short-term death from a car or industrial accidents and long-term injury from cardiovascular disease, obesity, and diabetes.

Step 7: Send a Thank You

After you've got a patient proper treatment like a PAP or an oral appliance, send a thank you note to the doctor who diagnosed them with UARS or OSA. Highlight how they've improved the patient's life, and mention that you hope to work with them in the future.

Thanking specialists serves two purposes. It expresses your appreciation so that they'll diagnose your future referrals, and it keeps your practice in their memory so that they'll choose you for their oral appliance patients. Remember, your goal for any of these professional relationships is a two-way referral stream.

Why Add Professionals Who Can't Diagnose to Your Referral Network?

It's important to also build connections with non-physicians like Occupational therapists, sleep and language pathologists, and myofunctional therapists. Why? Because getting your patients the therapy they need can improve their success with sleep apnea treatment, and because many of these professionals see adults whose eating and speaking issues are related to tongue and palate issues. When dentists and therapists focused on oral-motor issues work together, everyone's patients see better outcomes.

Building relationships with these professionals works much like building them with physicians. Outreach, education, and being friendly and approachable will help you build connections that get your patients and their patients the help that they need.

As I started referring patients, I realized that some of the physicians in my network would see my patients sooner, get them sleep studies sooner, and be more sympathetic to their reasons for not being able to comply with PAP treatment. So I started gravitating towards those offices, and we've gradually built stronger relationships. It was a lot easier and organic than I expected, but again, the key was just doing a good job with sleep medicine. That's how I earned the respect of other providers.

Roadblocks to Building Your Referral Network

A good relationship with area physicians is the first step to a successful sleep practice. What do you do when you're not getting anywhere? Why isn't anyone responding to your calls and emails? Why do your team members report that reaching out in person doesn't work? If you're hitting a roadblock on building a referral network, here are some hints that can help you out.

If You're in a Smaller Town or Suburb

If you're in a smaller town or suburb, you may face issues because most of your patients are used to leaving town for care. Building relationships with the local hospital may be difficult, because the most popular specialists are 45 minutes to an hour away, in bigger cities with more competitive referral networks.

In this case, try reaching out to your local PCPs instead. Maybe you need to connect with nurse practitioners if they're the group providing most of the day-to-day care in your town. It could also be helpful to talk to the hospital and practice administrators. In a situation where there's a local hospital but most people go to the bigger city for treatment, smaller hospitals are often looking for a way to "keep patients local." Partnering with them for your sleep dentistry program could help both your practice and their hospital.

If You're in a Bigger City

If you're finding that the physicians you approach already have preferred providers for sleep dentistry, you'll need to modify your list. Instead of going with older or more established physicians, look for people who are new to the area and only recently opened their practices, or people who are aggressively advertising that they're seeking new patients and trying to expand. Frankly, you don't need the oldest or most experienced physician to diagnose your UARS and OSA patients. You've already screened and examined them. In adults, it's very difficult to OVER-diagnose sleep breathing issues. If they failed the screenings, they need a sleep study. You just need someone who, in your state, is permitted to order one and interpret the results.

Younger, hungrier physicians are more eager to build the kind of relationships you want. Reach out to them. Give them a call or go visit. Talk about how you can help build each other's practices while improving your community's health.

Remembering the 7-Touch Rule of Marketing, and Other Hints

Remember when you were concerned about marketing your program? Here, building relationships with physicians, is where the marketing actually happens. You don't need billboards and newspaper ads to build your relationships with physicians, but you should consider a few principles of marketing:

- **It can take up to 7 marketing 'touches' to get a response** - So, meet people at educational events, send postcards and letters, call, email, visit, and...maybe you need one last contact to convince them to respond to you. Remember, your sleep program is a high priority to you, but it is not a high priority to the physicians. You need to build their sense of interest and urgency until it becomes important enough to act on.
- **Be an authority** - To partner with a physician, you need to convince them that you're serious about your program and sleep dentistry. Learn the science and medicine backing up your program. Be ready to talk about it. Get out in the community as a sleep evangelist so that you have a reputation as a serious practitioner of sleep medicine who cares about patient lives. Make it clear that you can pull your weight in this partnership, you're not just along for the ride.
- **Be likeable** - People want to partner with people they like. So be friendly and warm. Be helpful. Be considerate and willing to say "thank you for your help." You can even ask for advice. You want your physician network to be happy when they hear from you. If you're unsure how to do this without going too far and becoming an annoyance, ask a good friend for advice.
- **Leverage reciprocity** - People are hard-wired to reciprocate favors. So, send a little swag (like note pads). Send over a few test referrals. Invite your prospective physicians to

educational luncheons where you provide the food. Drop off treats for their office teams along with your contact info.

I know we all got into this field to become excellent clinicians and to improve our communities. Building these relationships can feel strange and uncomfortable – we're dentists, not realtors or drug reps. Even if you're nervous, keep working on these person-to-person connections. They're what you have to do now so that you can save lives down the road.

Implementation on Target!

After this chapter you should:

- Make your list of potential specialists and get their contact info
- Make the first contact with at least 3 specialists and follow up appropriately
- Identify your roadblocks to referrals and start to remove them
- Have at least one person you can work with to get your patients sleep studies

8. Setting Up Your Sleep Funnels in the Practice

In this chapter, you'll learn:

- What an office sleep funnel is
- How your team can help
- Electronic and print resources for your funnel
- Which screening support your funnel
- Why authority marketing is an important part of your funnel
- How to clear roadblocks to your sleep funnel

Good relationships with area physicians are essential to your sleep practice, but you also need patients who are excited about and interesting in sleep dentistry. In my own practice, existing patients are an endless source of new sleep dentistry patients.

Why? Because even if a patient doesn't suffer from sleep-disordered breathing, someone they know does. They have spouses, partners, parents, and children who snore or choke in their sleep. They have coworkers who are flummoxed about their inability to lose weight and friends who worry about a new diagnosis of high blood pressure.

People your patients love are suffering from poor sleep breathing, and your patients are worried about them but don't know how to help. When you set up sleep funnels in your office that inform your patients about your sleep dentistry program, you give them the tools they need to help their friends, family, and coworkers.

I tried to leap into sleep dentistry too quickly. My first few patients, I sprung sleep dentistry on them without warning, and they were annoyed. They were expecting a talk about teeth, not all of this other stuff. So I learned my lesson. Part of educating people is preparing them to learn. A tennis instructor doesn't randomly ambush children on the street and make them work on their backhands. And I couldn't ambush patients, even to save their lives. I needed to set up a funnel.

What Do Funnels Have to Do With Sleep Breathing?

So, what is a funnel? In marketing, a funnel is a pathway that takes people from a broad idea about a brand or product to a specific decision. For instance, you visit the "Joe's Shoe Shack" just to see what products are in stock. The site might have a banner up top "Our new 2022 boots are in stock and selling out fast." Ooh. Suddenly boots sound interesting. Why don't you click and see what styles they have? It won't take a minute. "Search by color!" the site proclaims.

You're still mostly playing around, but you've always sort of wanted a pair of blue boots, so you search and...15 minutes later, your order is placed, your stylish new blue boots are on the way, and you have experienced a funnel. You started with a broad expectation and no plans and ended with a specific decision.

Other people might not have stuck with the funnel as long as you did. They might have taken a quick look and found nothing of interest, clicked through but thought "maybe for Christmas," or put a pair of shoes in the cart but never completed the checkout.

A sleep funnel is similar, but you're not trying to sell the patient on a pair of shoes. Instead, you want to take them from wondering what sleep dentistry is to letting you solve their SDB problems. Not every patient will go all the way through the funnel, just as not every visitor to "Joe's Shoe Shack" will complete a purchase.

Every office sleep funnel is different because every practice is different. However, the most successful ones have most or all of the following features:

- Team members who talk about sleep dentistry
- Reading material in the waiting area to promote healthy sleep
- Posters in the bathrooms, patient operatories, and waiting area
- Basic sleep and health screening for all patients at least once a year
- Videos about sleep dentistry in the waiting area
- "Ask us about sleep dentistry" swag
- Sleep medicine certifications and memberships on the walls
- Refer a friend sleep dentistry cards
- QR codes that direct to a sleep dentistry page on the website
- Occasional email blasts about sleep dentistry, once or twice a year

The basic principles of a good sleep funnel are multiple touches, some sort of written commitment (like a screening or a referral card), and education that explains the *why* of sleep breathing. Let's look at each part of the office sleep funnel and how it gets patients excited about your sleep program.

Getting the Team Talking About Sleep Dentistry

In Chapter 5 we talked about how to get your team excited about sleep dentistry and on board with the process. Now, we're going to give them opportunities to interact with patients about sleep dentistry. When you start, your team will only have a theoretical relationship with sleep dentistry. They've learned a little about it, they're excited, they're willing to talk about the program.

As time goes on this should change. There will be people on your team who have SDB, or who have family members with SDB. You'll help them or their family and friends get treatment. Then their message will become more personal and even more compelling. It will stop being, "This is a good thing we're doing in the office" and become, "This changed my life and could change yours."

In the meantime, as a patient moves through the office, here are a few places that your team can nudge them so that they'll be ready to think about sleep dentistry:

- **At the pre-appointment call or text** - Appointment reminders should include a notice like "We're now offering sleep dentistry! If you snore or experience daytime sleepiness, we can help!"
- **At check-in** - When the patient checks in, the front desk should let them know that there will be a sleep screening since the office now offers sleep dentistry services.
- **On the way back to the room** - The patient can hear more about sleep dentistry and why it matters.
- **During the hygiene appointment** - Hygienists can incorporate talk about sleep with their other conversation during cleanings.
- **When they see you** - By the time you talk to a patient, they'll be primed to hear about sleep.
- **At checkout** - If you ask for referrals and offer referral cards, ask specifically for friends or family who could benefit from sleep dentistry.

Having the team talk about sleep doesn't mean ONLY talking about sleep – that's scripted and unnatural. But remember the "7 touches" theory of marketing? Every mention is a"'touch" that makes your patient more curious about sleep dentistry. You're starting to break through the wall of denial –"Everyone snores! I'm fine! All moms fall asleep at the wheel sometimes!" and getting the patients to a place where you can help them feel better and get healthier.

What Kind of Reading Material in the Waiting Room Promotes Healthy Sleep?

Before you select reading material, think about who sits in your waiting room, and for how long? Are patients there while they fill out forms? Are parents sitting in the waiting room during their children's appointments? Are most people on their phones, or do they sometimes flip through the magazines and brochures? With that in mind, try a selection of:

- **Books about healthy sleep** - Put a sticker on the cover that says "Loaner Copy," and include your contact info. People can't read a whole book in the waiting room, but they may take a copy home, share it, and bring it back later. Keep a stash and replace them as necessary.
- **Magazine articles with sleep and health themes** - If you receive some provider-focused publications, it's OK to put these out there. Otherwise, you may need to have reprints out, since not every wellness magazine talks about sleep every month.
- **Brochures about sleep medicine topics.**
- **QR codes that link to sleep articles patients can read on their phones.**

Even if people don't pick up and read the materials, they'll see the titles and recognize that your practice takes good sleep seriously – and they may ask your team why a dentist cares so much about sleep.

Do Posters and Flyers Do Any Good?

They do if you put them where people have nothing else to look at! Posters in the bathrooms can get a great response because bathrooms are boring. You can also attach them to the plexiglass near the front desk, and place them in the patient operatories. When people are bored, they look at things. Let some of those things educate patients about sleep!

Adding a Sleep and Wellness Screening

An annual sleep and wellness screening is an essential part of your sleep funnel. You already complete oral cancer screens and regular x-rays. At every appointment, you ask about updates to the patient's health history. Now, you should ensure that every patient receives a sleep and blood pressure screening at least once a year.

You should also look closely at the health updates. Is a patient now diagnosed with or taking drugs used to treat high blood pressure, type 2 diabetes, prediabetes, or metabolic syndrome? Any new diagnoses of these conditions should trigger a fresh sleep screen and also a sleep study.

Have a team member explain why the sleep screenings are important. Sleep directly impacts oral health because OSA can cause tooth grinding and TMJ. However, the impact on whole-body health from OSA is your main concern, and if OSA is causing issues like hypertension or diabetes, your office is here to help.

Some offices have the patients fill out the screenings, others have the patients work with a dental assistant. Find out what works for you, but get every patient screened at least once a year and whenever their health status changes.

Having patients fill out the screening ahead of their appointments, with a letter explaining what it was, helped a lot. So did brochures and posters in the waiting room. Little nudges got them thinking about SDB long before I entered the room.

Put Screens to Good Use

Do you have screens in the patient operatories and the waiting room? It's fine to turn them to a patient-chosen program during the cleaning, but the rest of the time, put those screens to work for your office. In a well-run office, patients won't be in the waiting room or sitting alone in the chair for very long. That means you can use those few, precious moments for patient education.

Create videos of you or a team member talking about sleep and sleep dentistry, and let them loop. I recommend getting a local videographer to help with these – no one wants to watch an amateurish video. Taking the time to present yourself well makes it easier to educate your patients.

What Do You Mean by "Sleep Dentistry Swag?"

Anything that says "Ask us about Sleep Dentistry" will help prime the patients and invite conversation. These can be buttons for your team to wear on their uniforms, sleep dentistry branding on the pens they use to fill out forms, or even sleep masks in their dental 'treat' bags. All of these little reminders help them associate your practice with sleep and make it more likely that they'll speak up and ask about the sleep issues in their family. Remember that the goal of your sleep funnels is to prepare people for screening, make them eager for a diagnosis and treatment, and get them excited about getting help for their family and friends. Education and enthusiasm help, but these little reminders keep the idea fresh in their heads so that they don't forget the moment that they leave your chair.

Your Walls Can Give You Authority

Why do marketers and practice experience experts tell you to hang your successes on the walls of your office? Because it's effective! Your patients want to know that you're good at what you do and that you keep getting better.

With that in mind, get some of your sleep-related certifications framed, and hang them in the waiting room. If your local paper has covered your sleep dentistry launch, hang that up there too! I know it can feel a bit like bragging, but to reach your patients, push at the edges of your comfort zone and announce your sleep medicine achievements, even if they don't feel that significant to you.

Start a Sleep Referral Avalanche

Why do referrals prime patients to say "yes" to sleep medicine? Because so many of us are more concerned about our family's health than we are about our own. I see it over and over in my practice.

A mother will bring her teen daughter in, concerned about sleep breathing issues. As we go over her symptoms and screening results, the teen will grow increasingly irritated. Finally, she blurts out, "I don't know why we're here for me. Mom is *much* worse than I am!"

So many of our patients put their own healthcare last. They'll move heaven and earth to get help for their spouses and kids, but they let their own SDB go untreated until they're in crisis. Referring family and friends creates circumstances where the referrer also accepts treatment.

With that in mind, start asking patients for sleep referrals! When you go through the sleep screen you can ask if the screening triggered concerns about any friends or family. Have two-part referral cards handy (so that you have one for your records and the patient has one to pass on), and encourage spouses and partners to accompany one another to the screening appointments. Sleep medicine changes lives, and getting your patients to think about who else it could help is a step towards getting them to accept care for themselves.

QR Codes Can Help Patients Go Deeper

Some of your patients will be bored by the idea of sleep medicine. Some of your patients will be excited, and eager to find out more. Make it easy for them! Have places around the office where a short sentence or two about some aspect of sleep medicine is presented with a QR code that links to a longer, publicly available article. People who just want the short facts can read the two-line summary, people who want to go deeper can scan the code and read the link. This is a low-cost, easy way to reach more of your patients and nudge them towards treatment.

Keep Your Email/Newsletter Group in the Loop

Do patients read the emails from your office? Some do. Others just read the headline. Both groups benefit if you add occasional posts on sleep dentistry to your usual round of news and marketing. Remember, it can take seven touches for an idea to sink in and for a person to take action. Most of your patients only come in once or twice a year. Nudges from your emails help prepare them to say yes to sleep dentistry!

Roadblocks to a Great Funnel

Many practices encounter roadblocks while setting up funnels. Here are a few frequent issues that we see, and how to solve them.

My Patients Are Surprised and Irritated When We Ask Them to Fill Out a Sleep Screening Form At Check-In

You may want to put a little more effort into your funnel BEFORE they arrive in the office. That means having the sleep forms available as a download with your new patient forms and making sure that all reminders such as texts, calls, and postcards, mention your new sleep screening program.

If the issue is that your patients don't want to fill out another form in the waiting room, consider having a dental assistant give them an oral screening or having patients fill out the form in the hygienist's chair before the appointment begins.

No One Seems Interested in Sleep Dentistry When I See Them.

If your patients aren't at all interested in sleep breathing when you see them, this is an issue with your team. Your team may need to practice talking about sleep and answering patient questions. Maybe you need to take time to role-play or bring in friends and family without dental knowledge so that you can see if the team is talking in ways that patients can understand.

People Keep Taking My Loaner Books and Not Bringing Them Back, but I Don't Know *Who* is Taking Them.

Loaner books can help people talk to their family and friends about sleep, and they can persuade your patients to get diagnosed and treated. On the other hand, it's helpful to know *who* is borrowing, or taking the books. If your office is concerned that books are walking out the door and never coming back, try a different strategy. Have books in the waiting room with a note that states "If you'd like a copy to continue reading at home or to share with family and friends, ask at the desk!" Then get the contact information for these people before you give them a book to take home. And always, always, make sure every book has a sticker with your office's information.

I'm Not Getting Any Referrals From My Patients.

If you're not getting any sleep dentistry referrals from the referral card, you don't have a sleep funnel problem. You have a patient engagement and referral problem. Delegate one of your office team to read up on best practices for asking for, and getting referrals from your sleep patients. There are hundreds of good, solid articles on patient referrals for dental offices because it's one of the most powerful tools for bringing new patients into the practice.

I Hate Being on Camera! I Don't Want to Make Videos.

Videos aren't everyone's talent. If you don't want to star in your office sleep dentistry videos, talk to your team! You probably have at least one person in your office who's a great communicator and loves the camera. Then you can appear in the videos in candid working footage instead of having to be the main face and voice.

Setting up good sleep funnels is an important step to building a successful sleep dentistry practice. The best thing about in-office funnels is that they're easy to refresh and maintain. That leaves you more time to focus on the clinical part of sleep dentistry and helps your practice grow.

Once I got the right funnels in place, I didn't even have to bring up dental sleep medicine when I entered the room. The patients were asking me about it before I could even start talking! People need this. They just need a little bit of education to realize how much treating SDB will improve their lives.

Implementation on Target!

After this chapter, you should:

- Sketch out a plan for your sleep funnel
- Assign team members to help you create materials
- Plan any video resources
- Develop a list of good sleep books for your waiting room
- Identify potential roadblocks that your particular practice will face
- Choose your sleep screenings and how to administer them

9: OAT for Adults: A Quick Guide

In this chapter, you'll learn:

- **How to conduct an oral appliance exam**
- **The basics of a few different sleep appliances**
- **How to take impressions and use a George gauge**
- **How to structure your delivery appointment**
- **How follow-ups and titration will work**
- **How to prevent the most common complications of OAT**

There are two main modes of treatment when you're practicing adult sleep dentistry: you can refer to an MD for a PAP machine, or you can create a custom oral appliance. In general, most of your patients will want an oral appliance. Oral appliances are more versatile, more comfortable, and tend to have better compliance than PAP machines.

Here are the main steps to oral appliance therapy:

- A careful examination of the patient, including a complete dental history, future dental plans, and any allergies
- Choosing an appliance that meets the patient's needs
- Taking impressions for the appliance and, if necessary, a morning aligner
- Delivering the appliance

- Instructions on good sleep hygiene in conjunction with the appliance
- Follow-ups and titration

Don't rush through the process. Every successful treatment will give you a happy, healthy patient who goes out into the community and spreads the word about your life-changing sleep program. A well-fitting oral appliance that matches your patient's needs will seem like a miracle to them, so it's worth making a careful, well-considered decision and explaining it carefully to your patient.

My biggest piece of advice is not to be overwhelmed by all the choices for appliances out there. Every single appliance has positives and drawbacks. Familiarize yourself with several, and then choose what's best for each patient.

What to Look For in the Oral Appliance Exam

When a patient has an oral appliance appointment, they have already received a diagnosis of UARS or OSA. This examination is to help you determine an appropriate course of treatment. During the exam, record any:

- Existing restorations
- Tongue size, position
- Signs of bruxism
- Periodontal health
- Dentition health
- Missing teeth

Ask your patient about their dental plans. Are they planning to have more work done? Thinking about starting Invisalign? Because an oral appliance lasts 3-5 years, it's important to consider not just their teeth now, but how they are likely to change over the next several years. Some dental appliances work better with ongoing restorative dental work than others do.

Also, ask your patient about any allergies to materials like latex or acrylic, and about claustrophobia. How much space and movement do they need to feel comfortable? Remember, therapy for sleep apnea is only successful if your patients can comply with the treatment.

Choosing an Oral Appliance for Sleep Apnea

The first thing we need to understand is "How does an oral appliance, also known as a Mandibular Advancement Device (MAD) work?"

These appliances work by:

- Improving airway by repositioning the mandible
- Preventing the collapse of tongue base into the oropharynx
- Placing tension on pharyngeal musculature as well as stabilization to help support the airway thus preventing further collapse

There are more than 300 custom sleep apnea appliances approved for use in the United States. No one appliance will work for all of your patients.

Important points to consider when choosing an appliance:

- Is it adjustable? Does it allow for modification if dental treatment is needed?
- Can it be calibrated? Does it allow for vertical and/or horizontal movement to open the airway if needed?
- Is there posterior support? Does it stabilize the TMJ for patients that may need it?
- Does it allow movement of the mandible? Is there lateral freedom of movement in bruxers?
- What about lip seal? Will it help eliminate mouth breathing and allow nasal breathing?

- How much tongue space does it allow? One thing to keep in mind is the size and shape of a patient's tongue. Proper nighttime tongue position is essential for healthy sleep. If an appliance interferes with your patient's ability to rest their tongue on the roof of the mouth, it is not the best choice. We want to move that jaw forward and encourage a healthy tongue position for maximum effectiveness of OAT.
- How much tooth coverage does it allow to prevent tooth movement?

Attachment and propulsion mechanisms for oral appliances:

Attached:

- Midline traction
- Bilateral traction
- Bilateral compression

Unattached:

- Bilateral interlocking

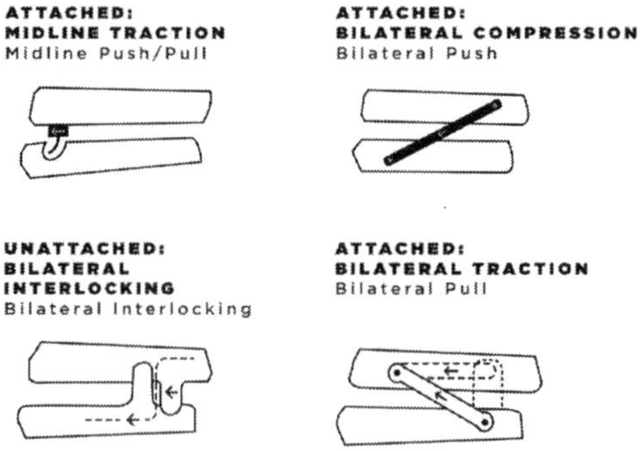

Image adapted from: https://idt.cdeworld.com/courses/5023-part-iii-oral-appliance-therapy-for-sleep-disordered-breathing

Here is an easier way of looking at how these work:

Considering that the maxilla is the stationary arch -

Traction -> anchoring on the maxilla and PULLING the mandible forward

Compression -> bracing against maxilla and PUSHING the mandible forward

Attached: Midline Traction

This is a "push/pull" type of appliance. Forces applied by the advancement mechanism or by mandibular closing affect the anterior teeth as do dislodging forces.

Examples of these types of appliances are TAP and Klearway.

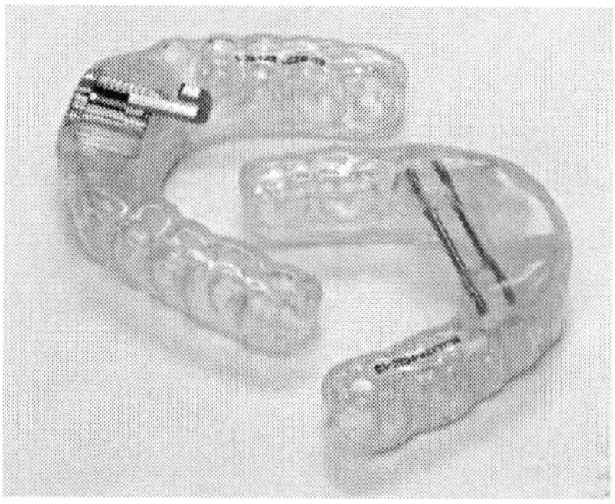

Tap Appliance

Attached: Bilateral Traction

This is a "pull" type appliance. Forces applied are focused on maxillary anterior teeth and/or bicuspids, mandibular posterior teeth.

Tip: Watch for non-retentive mandibular molars

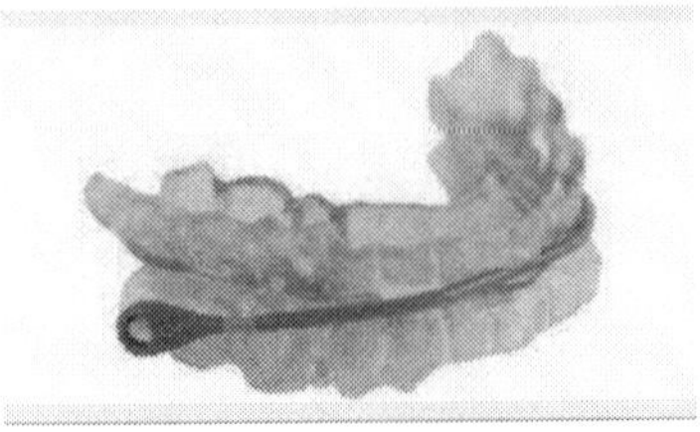

Somnomed Avant Appliance

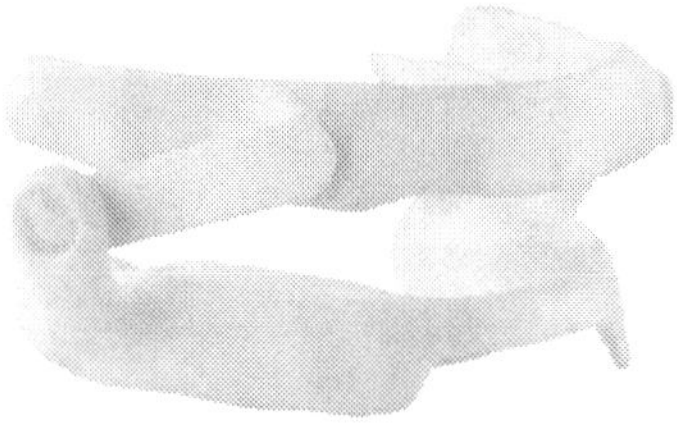

Panthera Appliance

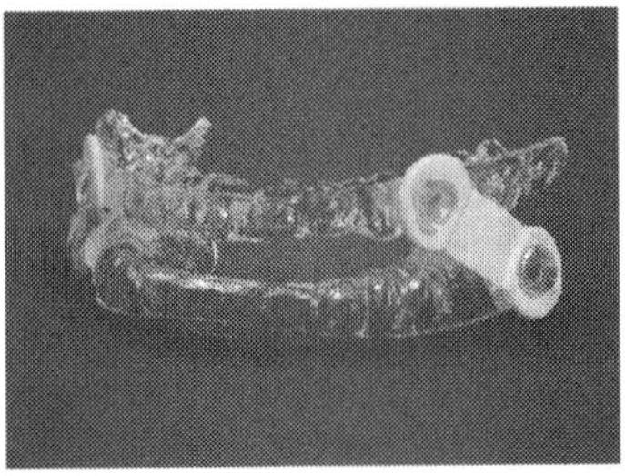

EMA Appliance

Attachment: Bilateral Compression

This is a "push" type appliance. Forces applied are focused on mandibular anterior and maxillary posterior teeth.

These appliances typically have a "propulsion-arm" mechanism.

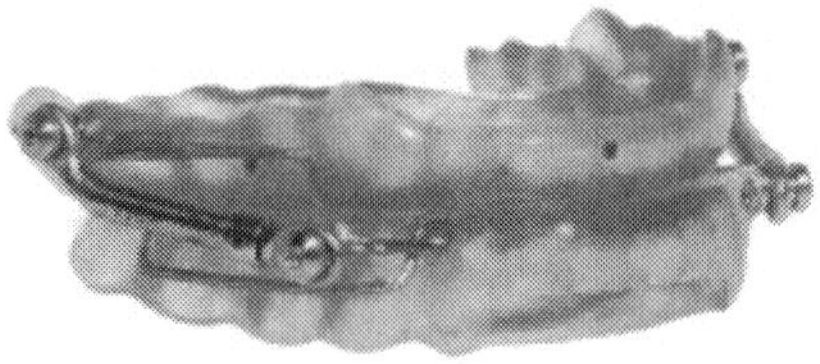

Herbst Appliance

Unattached: Bilateral Interlocking

This is a "push" type appliance. Forces applied are distributed along the maxillary and mandibular posterior teeth.

Examples: Any "dorsal" type appliance.

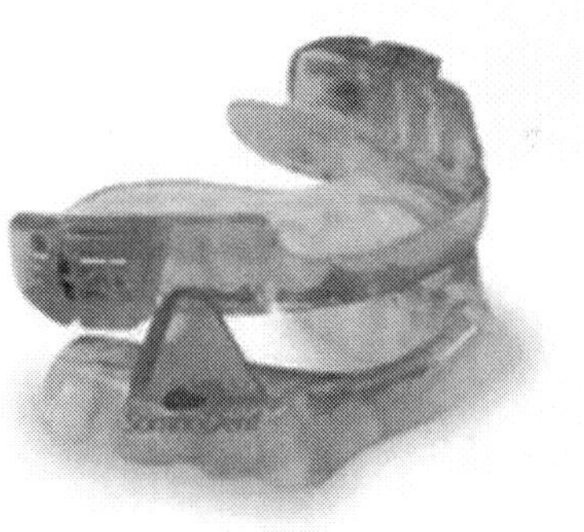

Somnodent Appliance

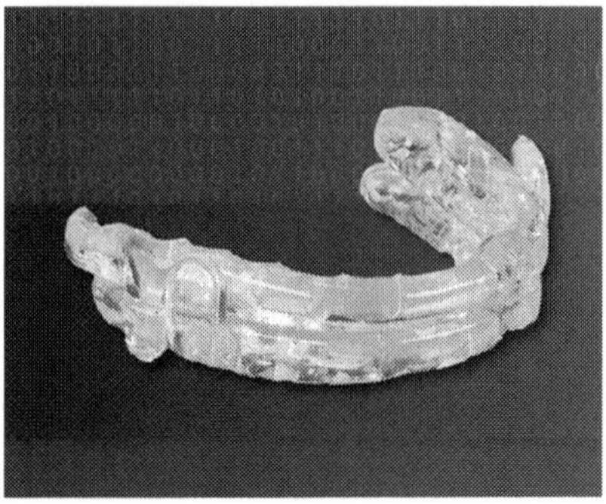

Prosomnus Appliance

Sometimes elastics may be needed with Attached Bilateral Compression or Unattached Bilateral Interlocking appliances. These help keep the mandible supported and protruded, lip seal, reduce mouth breathing, maintain a patent airway.

Keep in mind: Some patients have latex allergies. Have latex-free options available.

For retention decision in appliances, consider:

- flexion into available undercuts
- path of insertion and removal
- tooth angulation
- arch angulation
- clinical crown length

Temporary Appliances

I use temporary appliances for patients who are having a lot of restorative dental work done but need sleep apnea treatment during the process. It's also a good match for my Invisalign patients. It works with the aligners, and we can hold off on a permanent appliance until their teeth are in the final position.

My TAP

My TAP is a temporary appliance, which is easy to titrate. The upper and lower trays are submerged in warm water for a minute until they turn from white to clear. One at a time, they are then placed on the teeth. The adjustment dial is used to advance in 1/3mm increments as needed. It has a 23mm range of adjustment.

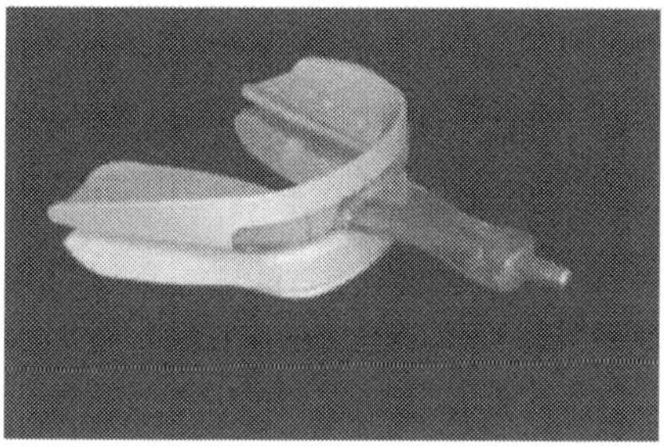

Blue Pro

The Blue Pro is another temporary thermoplastic appliance. Upper and lower trays are immersed in hot water until the material becomes clear. It is then cooled for a minute and fitted to the upper and lower arches. They are then connected to the appliance and reinserted to find the optimal level of mandibular protrusion.

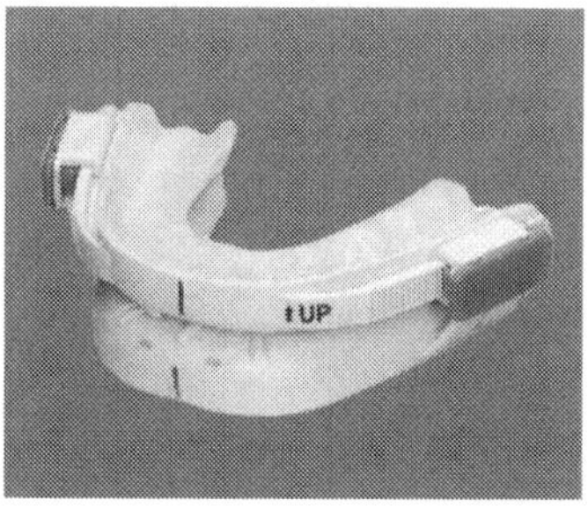

Silent Sleep

This appliance consists of a single-piece tray system that is customized to the patient's teeth using GC Reline, a chair-side vinyl polysiloxane.

This appliance is fitted to the posterior teeth of the patient while the patient is in a protrusive position.

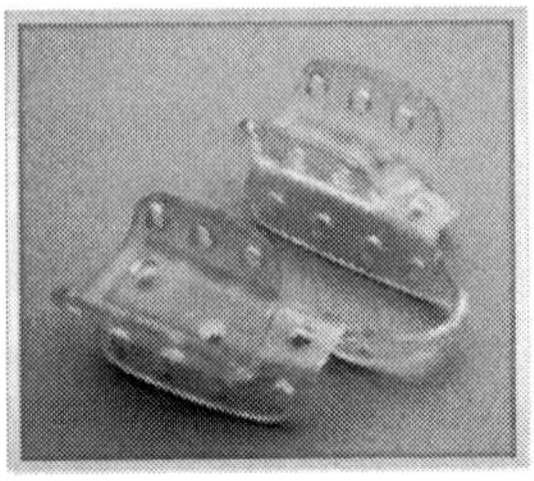

Somnodent Alpha

This appliance consists of 2 generic trays which fit over the upper and lower teeth. The lower tray is held in a protrusive position by an advancement mechanism.

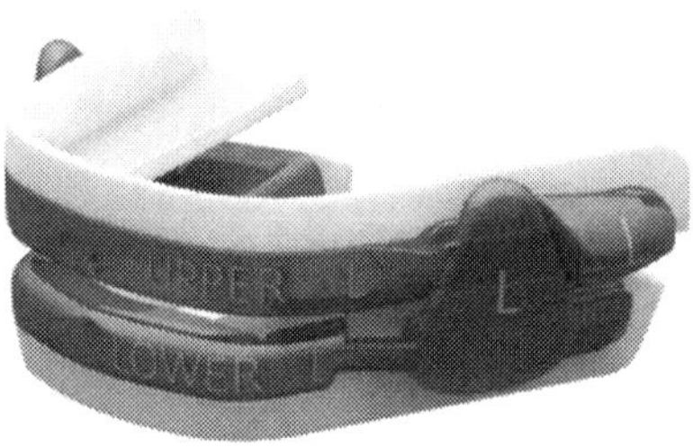

Most of the time, the first appliance I try with a patient works great. But occasionally, a specific appliance will turn out to be a bad fit. Maybe they just don't like how it feels, or maybe they have some small, oral quirk that makes a specific appliance unbearable when another feels fine. At this point, you may need to document the issues and start the process with insurers again. However, if someone has OSA, they need a treatment they can comply with. The health issues down the line are going to be much more expensive for them than having to get a different appliance.

Taking Impressions

The next step in getting the right oral appliance for your patient is taking impressions. The better your impressions, the better fit you'll get, and the better the fit the better the compliance with therapy and the results. Until recently, I used physical impressions in my office, but I've switched to digital. In this section, I'll outline both methods.

Over the years, I've used many different media for taking impressions. The one that I found worked best was a PVS material. These give me the best margins and details, so the appliances made from these impressions have a better fit. However, choose the medium that works best for you. If you're routinely getting bad fit on appliances, you may want to demo different media to see if you get better results from a different brand or supplier.

When taking impressions for a sleep appliance, make sure to get a good impression of the soft tissue as well as the hard tissue. If the patient has third molars, you will need to decide whether they should be included in the appliance design and what appliance will work best for them. The "standard" is a patient with no third molars since most people in the US have them removed as teens.

Whether you're using digital or physical impressions, you'll want upper, lower, and bite impressions. Because the bite impression is for how the appliance will advance the jaw, I use a George Gauge as part of the process.

In addition to standard impressions or scans, take photos of the patient from the front and sides, both open and closed-mouthed. Get occlusal views as well. These will be useful for comparison later, in case the patient worries that their teeth are moving or the shape of their face has changed. Good "before" pictures can help set minds at ease "after."

Finally, get a uvula shot, as this is useful for insurance documentation.

Using a George Gauge

After the impressions, you're going to need to get your patient's George Gauge number so that the sleep appliance can be designed and produced with the correct range of motion. Every patient's jaw moves differently. It is essential to take this measurement to get the correct fit.

If your office does not currently have a George Gauge and single-use bite forks, you can order them from www.greatlakesdentaltech.com. This measurement will make all the difference in fit, comfort, compliance, and results in your sleep dentistry patients.

There are a few things you can do to make it easier for your team to use this tool.

- Take the measurements and compute the readings on the first 10-12 patients yourself, with your team observing.
- Make a video of yourself doing this so that your team can watch and rewatch.
- When you record the readings, don't record the numbers as + and -. It will be easier for your team to complete the calculations if you list the protrusion number as P and the retrusion number as R.
- Keep a small pocket calculator in the operatory or imaging room, wherever you are taking impressions.
- The formula that I use for the George Gauge number is .7(p+r)-r = GG#.
- If .7(p+r) is a decimal, round. For instance, 6.01 to 6.49 rounds down to 6, 6.5 to 6.99 rounds up to 7.
- Keep in mind that some of your team may not have done math in a while, so have them practice this a lot.

Choosing the Bite Fork

The George Gauge comes with a 2mm, 3mm, and 5mm bite fork. Start with the 2mm fork and check to see if the patient has at least a

4mm space between their upper and lower molars on each side. A 4mm space is the minimum needed for the lab to make an appliance based on their bite impressions. If the space on either side is too small, use a 5mm fork instead.

Steps for Finding the George Gauge Number

Here is a step-by-step guide for finding the George Gauge Number. You may want to hang a laminated copy in the areas where you take impressions.

1. Place the bite fork in the mouth.
2. Make sure the fork is set to 0. If it is not zeroed before you start measuring your GG number will be off and the finished appliance will not fit correctly.
3. Have the patient move their lower jaw forward as far as possible. Record the measurement as P for Protrusion.
4. Have the patient move their lower jaw back as far as possible. Record the measurement as R for Retrusion.
5. Add R+P.
6. Multiply this number by .7. This is Y
7. If necessary, round Y.
8. Subtract R from Y . This is your GG number for the patient.

Example 1:

The patient's P number is 7 and her R number is 2.

- P+R =9
- .7(9) = 6.3
- 6.3 rounds down to 6.
- 6-R = 6-2 =4.
- The GG # is 4

Example 2:

The patient's P number is 6 and his R number is 2

- P+R = 8
- .7(8) = 5.6
- 5.6 rounds up to 6
- 6-2 =4
- The GG # is 4

Have your team practice these calculations using real measurements – you can have them measure and calculate for each other!

Why .7 instead of .5 or .6?

In my years making oral appliances for sleep therapy, I've found that 70% is the best setting for the appliance. It achieves maximum benefit quickly, and with very little titration or discomfort. Some sleep dentists prefer to be more conservative and to start at 50% or 60%, but I find that these lower settings mean more titration visits and a longer time before the patient starts seeing results. If patients don't see results quickly, compliance falls off and they will decide OAT just didn't work for them.

If you'd rather start at 50% or 60%, replace .7 with .5 or .6 in the formula above and in the steps for finding the George Number.

Taking the Bite Impressions With the George Gauge

Once you have computed the George number, use the bite fork to take impressions. Set the fork to the George number. If you are taking physical impressions you can either remove the fork from the mouth and cover the disposable part with media, or spread the media in the mouth while the fork is in place. Neither is better, it's just a matter of personal preference. Choose the procedure that gives you and your team the best impressions.

If you're using digital imaging, you can cut the fork and use the bite scan to scan the bite. The lab will use this information to correctly align the upper and lower parts of the oral appliance.

My team was a little nervous about the George Gauge at first, so I took time to demonstrate it, teach them, and have them try it on each other. With a little practice, they could handle this part of the appointment easily. At every step of implementation, there was a place where I had to tell my team, "You don't think you can learn this new thing, but I know you can, and you'll be great!" Once they know you have confidence in them, your team will rise to the occasion.

Appliance Delivery

After you send the order for the appliance to the lab, your work is done for a while. Your next contact with this patient will be when the appliance arrives in your office. Will you schedule an appointment to pick up the appliance at the imaging appointment, or will you simply call when it arrives? Do not let the patient leave your office without making sure that they understand when and how they will be contacted for pick-up.

At the delivery appointment, you will:

- Have the patient try the appliance on
- Check for sore spots
- Create the AM aligner and instruct the patient in its use
- Teach the patient how to clean the appliance
- Have the patient practice placing and removing the appliance a few times while you watch
- Have the patient practice cleaning the appliance
- Talk to the patient about their experiences
- Discuss side effects
- Make an appointment for follow-up care

During this appointment, how you talk to the patient can influence their compliance with the therapy plan. Your patient has come to the chair with pre-conceptions and is forming ideas about the appliance. Try asking "How does it feel? Is it what you expected? Is it more or less obtrusive than you expected?"

Let the patients talk to you about their expectations, and be reassuring. By talking about feelings and expectations, you take the focus off the appliance and put it on their experiences. This increases their compliance with treatment because the appliance is not some alien invader, it's a choice they made for themselves.

I always warn our patients to expect excessive saliva for the first few days, until their body adjusts to having the appliance in their mouth at night. They need to know that this is normal so that they don't give up on the treatment plan.

Creating the AM Aligner

Our patients must wear their aligners for 30 minutes every morning to help bring their bite into the "daytime position." After a night of the jaw thrust forward, they need the aligner to help their muscles to return to normal.

For our morning aligners, I use thermoplastic from Patterson Dental, but you can also order from Great Lakes. Some brands of appliances also offer a morning aligner option.

Remember, the aligner is just there to help the patient guide their jaw back to the proper position after a night of therapy.

Sleep Hygiene Information

When people aren't breathing well in their sleep, they develop bad habits. They have a harder time staying awake during the day because their bodies can't do the work of sleep. They can't fall asleep easily at night because their brain associates sleep with "almost dying over and over again." We've gotten them the appliance that will ameliorate their sleep breathing issues, now we need to help them break their bad sleep-related habits as well.

At appliance delivery, give your patients a handout about good sleep hygiene, and go over the following points:

- **No blue light in the bedroom** - Replace any Blue LED bulbs with yellow ones. Ban screens from the bedroom. If you want to read ebooks before bed, use an e-ink product like the Kindle Paperwhite, not a tablet or phone.
- **Go to bed at the same time every night, and make sure it's at least 8 hours before your wake-up time** - It's tempting to do one last thing, and then another last thing, and put off bed. Sleep is important work, too. Don't put it off.
- **Use a white noise machine if the background noises at home bother you**
- **Take a hot bath or shower before bed**
- **Keep your room 68 degrees or less**
- **Do not drink caffeine after 3 pm** - Because our patients have gotten used to excessive daytime sleepiness, many lean on caffeine to get through the afternoon and evening hours. Now that they're going to be breathing, they should cut the caffeine for better sleep.
- **No alcohol for 2 hours before bed** - Alcohol can depress your sleep breathing and disrupt your sleep cycles. Save it for early evening, not bedtime.
- **Learn how exercise affects your sleep** - If exercising before bed leaves you wide awake, move your workout to the morning. If it helps you get to sleep, then you can keep it in the evening.
- **Beds are for sleep and sex only** - If you work or watch TV in bed, your brain won't want to sleep there.
- **Avoid large meals or spicy food for 2 hours before bed** - Heartburn reduces sleep quality, and eating too close to bedtime can trigger heartburn.
- **Try sleep positioners** - A bed wedge or side sleeper can help patients choose positions that enhance sleep breathing and comfort.
- **Use Breathe Right strips or Nose Cones/Mutes to relearn nasal breathing**
- **Download a sleep tracking app to see how you sleep and if you're still snoring**

When you help patients develop good sleep habits, you increase their compliance with OAT and help them get more out of the device.

It might feel a little silly to give advice on sleep hygiene at first, but our patients need this. Often, no medical professional has ever talked to them about sleep and how to get more of it. When you practice Dental Sleep Medicine you're often the only provider in the patient's life teaching them these things!

Follow-ups and Titration

At appliance delivery, you'll schedule follow-up appointments. It can be helpful to schedule the first year's worth of follow-up all at once. Keep in mind that any appointments in the first month are included in the cost of the appliance, and so cannot be charged to the medical insurer. After that, all other follow-ups are charged. Your follow-up schedule should be:

- Two weeks after delivery
- One month after delivery
- Three months after delivery
- Six months after delivery
- One year after delivery
- Annual check-up
- Other appointments as needed

Again, schedule the two-week, one-month, three-month, six-month, and one-year appointments at the time of delivery. If you let the patient wait to make these, they may forget, and problems can develop with their bite, jaw, or tooth position. The way to get excellent compliance and results from OAT is to ensure that you and the patient are proactive about dealing with any bumps in the road.

Two-Week Appointment Checklist

At the two-week appointment, you will:

- Remind the patient to wear the morning aligner.
- Check to see if any sore spots need adjustments.
- Remind the patient how to clean the device.
- Ask how they're feeling, and if they've seen a difference.
- Answer any questions or concerns.
- Ask "On nights that you couldn't wear the device, what caused you to leave it out?" You can help them troubleshoot and remind them that the more they wear it, the healthier they'll be and the better they'll feel.

One-Month Appointment Checklist

At the one-month appointment, you will:

- Remind the patient to wear the morning aligner.
- Check to see if any sore spots need adjustments.
- Remind the patient how to clean the device.
- Teach the patient to titrate the device.
- Warn the patient not to titrate too quickly.
- Ask how they're feeling, and if they've seen a difference.
- Answer any questions or concerns.
- Ask "On nights that you couldn't wear the device, what caused you to leave it out?" You can help them troubleshoot and remind them that the more they wear it, the healthier they'll be and the better they'll feel.

3, 6, and 12-month, and Annual Appointment Checklists

At these follow-ups, you will

- Have the patient complete a new ESS to document any changes to daytime sleepiness.

- Order a home sleep test (HST) if permitted by your state. Otherwise, ask one of your physician-partners to order a sleep study.
- Check weight, BP, and neck circumference.
- Remind the patient to wear the morning aligner.
- Check to see if any sore spots need adjustments.
- Remind the patient how to clean the device.
- Ask how they're feeling, and if they've seen a difference.
- Answer any questions or concerns.
- Ask "On nights that you couldn't wear the device, what caused you to leave it out?" You can help them troubleshoot and remind them that the more they wear it, the healthier they'll be and the better they'll feel.

When I started, I was worried a lot about complications. What if I gave someone TMJ? What if I made their bruxism worse? As I practiced, I realized that as long as the appliance was properly adjusted, the patients were free of pain and seeing great results.

Common Complications and How to Prevent and Treat Them

As doctors, we're often more worried than the patients about complications for OAT. However, we need the patient's buy-in to catch complications before they become serious. Remind your patients to call if they are noticing any changes to bite, any jaw pain, or any tooth movement. With any of these complications, we can correct them early on with minor adjustments to the appliance, but if they're allowed to continue for 6 months or a year, they can be much more difficult to treat and also impact a patient's ability to comply with therapy.

Diagnosing and Treating the Causes of Jaw Pain

When you're talking to a patient about jaw pain, the first step is to ask them to point to where the pain is worst. This will let you see whether it is joint pain or muscle pain. If the pain is up by their ear, it's usually a TMJ issue, but if it's in the cheek or temple, you are dealing with muscle pain.

For Joint Pain

The most common cause is a shift in the midline of the appliance. If it's shifted to the left, there will be worse pain in the left side, if it's shifted to the right there will be more pain in the right side. Adjust the appliance to even out the protrusion and bring the midline back to the center.

Do not immediately adjust the appliance backward. This is rarely the problem. It's more likely that it's not holding the jaw far enough forwards, and that the patient is still having apneas that cause clenching and grinding.

Ask the patient how they are sleeping and if they are snoring. If they are waking tired and still snoring, the appliance needs to be titrated forward to reduce clenching and grinding.

If the patient has stopped snoring and is waking refreshed, you can look into moving the appliance slightly backward to see if that helps.

For Muscle Pain

The most common cause of muscle pain is problems with the vertical direction of the appliance. If the appliance has posterior support, reduce the vertical a bit to relieve the pain. If the appliance has *no* vertical support (for instance, a TAP), then add an acrylic piece to give vertical support.

Continued Snoring

Sometimes, after treatment, patients continue to snore. Ask them how they feel when they wake, and take a close look at their ESS scores. If they're still experiencing daytime sleepiness, you'll need to move the appliance further forward. If, however, they are waking full of energy, they may be experiencing nasal snoring. These are the patients who can benefit from Breathe Right strips or nasal cones. If these don't stop the snoring, refer them to an ENT who can look for structural issues or who can treat allergies.

Bite Changes

Warn your patients at the beginning of treatment and at each subsequent appointment to be aware that bite changes are possible with OAT. The best way to prevent these is faithful use of the morning aligner, but some patients do report that they can correct their own bite without an aligner. If patients are concerned about bite changes and not using the aligner, the answer is to make it a habit.

Tooth Movement

Be sure to inform your patients to be alert to tooth movement. We most often see this with the first and second molars. If your patient flosses, it will help them notice when teeth are moving.

The best way to deal with tooth movement is to prevent it. The bottom piece of the appliance should be long enough to cover the distal of the second molar. Write this into your prescription. Sometimes, despite what you wrote, the lab will send an appliance that does not extend to the second molar. In this case, you have two options. You can make an acrylic piece in-house for the appliance, or you can send the appliance back and ask them to remake it.

If you make your own add-on, go back to the original models before treatment. You can also make an Essix retainer for them to wear during the day to shift the teeth back.

Sometimes, the device itself may be causing the tooth to shift. Is a sharp and pointy embrasure acting as a wedge and pushing the teeth apart? Grind it down. Is a ball clasp the culprit? Adjust it with pliers.

Remind your patients that being proactive by flossing and calling the office is their best defense against tooth movement. If they suspect movement, they must call immediately so that you can reverse it. If they let it go on too long, they may have to see an orthodontist.

Many dentists hold back from offering their patients OAT because they are worried about side effects. However, the side effects of OAT are easily preventable and are less severe than complications from untreated OSA. Remember, we are offering our patients the best alternative to PAP therapy out there. So many people avoid necessary sleep studies and diagnoses because they don't want to be stuck on a PAP for the rest of their lives. For them, OAT is literally lifesaving, and you are the only person who can offer it to your patients.

Implementation on Target!

After this chapter, you should:

- Research and demo sleep appliances and find your favorites
- Purchase a George Gauge and forks, and practice using them
- Teach your team to do the George Gauge math
- Plan how long the initial, delivery, and follow-up appointments will take, and start creating schedule blocks for them
- Develop a plan for treating complications

10: Follow Up/Outreach – Share Your Successes

In this chapter you will learn:

- **Why sharing your successes is the best internal and external marketing**
- **Ways to share successes and get your patients and team excited about sleep dentistry**
- **How to keep your own morale up, even when adding a new service is a steep learning curve**

Sometimes, as practitioners, we're too shy about our achievements. We come in. We do a good, thorough job. We change a patient's life, but we don't brag, even to our families. After all, we're dentists. We're careful, we strive for clinical excellence, and we get our patients smiling again. It's just part of the job.

Sharing stories about the lives we've changed seems grandiose. It's as if we were letter carriers bragging "I did a really good job with my deliveries today and got every piece of mail to the right person!" It feels egotistical to brag about doing what we're supposed to do. If we weren't changing lives and saving smiles, we'd just be terrible at our jobs.

If you want to succeed in sleep dentistry, you're going to have to get over this reticence about sharing your success stories. The biggest motivator for your sleep patients is going to be the hope you can give them. Hope increases the odds that they'll agree to a much-needed sleep study. It increases the chances that they'll say 'yes' to life-saving treatment after their diagnosis. And hope is what will get them through the early days of OAT, where the thing in their mouth feels funny and they're not sure that they'll see results.

Don't be afraid to share your wins! A life changed by sleep dentistry is something worth celebrating. You're helping people get healthy, and giving them true, lasting improvement in their lives. So don't be shy. The more you share, the more people you can help!

So many of the sleep patients I see have given up hope of a better life. They're resigned to being unhappy, unhealthy, and unrested. "It's just bad genes," they tell me. "I'm just getting old. I can't expect to live life without pain and heart problems." "My body has turned against me." Because no one has explained the underlying cause of their issues, and that this underlying cause is treatable with proven therapies, they've stopped looking for answers. Why should they get their hope up when they'll just be disappointed again?

You can restore hope. As you treat sleep patients and see their biomarkers improve, their energy levels recover, and the smiles return to their faces, you need to document your cases. Not just in terms of insurance, but so that you can have evidence for your next patients, the ones nervous about giving sleep medicine a chance.

In this chapter, I'm going to share some of my favorite ways to give a shout-out to your sleep successes. You don't have to use all of these or any of them. Some of these are things I do in my office, others are things that friends and students have done. You can find your own, personal way to spread the word and encourage your patients to get help. Take these as suggestions, and see if any give you ideas!

Video Testimonials, Short and Long

Video testimonials from existing patients are one of the most powerful tools there are to motivate new patients to accept treatment and to remind yourself and your team that the struggle is worth it and that you're changing and saving lives with sleep dentistry.

Get both short and long testimonials from some of your happiest patients, with permission to share. Your practice website, monitors in the office, YouTube, TikTok, Facebook, and Instagram Reels are all great places to share these videos. (Keep in mind that different sites are optimized for different video lengths!). Your patients want to know that you're helping people just like them.

A bonus is that the patients starring in the videos will share them with family and friends who also need these life-saving services. A little video goes a long way towards spreading the word about how sleep dentistry can help change lives.

Posts With Photos

These are a favorite in my practice. When you see someone for a follow-up, snap a picture of the new, healthy them. With permission, post these photos on social media. It's great for your patients to see that you're regularly changing lives with sleep dentistry and that even young and seemingly healthy people can have UARS and benefit from an appliance.

Case Study Book With Pictures and Short Stories

Many practices have success with these books, which you can have made on a site like Mixbooks. These books give patients something to look through while they wait in the waiting room or the chair. Keep the stories short and sweet, along the lines of:

Anna was always tired and draggy, but what mother of a three-year-old isn't? She joked that her life ran on caffeine. She was never without a large tea or coffee, and she relied on them to stay awake during her long commute. When she got home at night, she was exhausted and achy, but she kept pushing herself. Mornings were a mess of headaches and exhaustion. Surely things would get better once her daughter was a bit older?

After being diagnosed with UARS and getting an appliance, Anna couldn't believe the difference. Suddenly she could drive without nodding off. She still had energy at the end of the day and cut back on caffeine – not intentionally, but just because she stopped needing it. Her daughter can still outrun her – she is three, after all – but now Anna can make it through bedtime, and has the energy after to talk to her husband and indulge in hobbies. "It's amazing how such a small piece of plastic totally changed my life," Anna says, "I wish I had gotten into the office sooner!"

Pair each story with a picture, either a snapshot from an appointment or a nice family shot submitted by the patient. These sorts of photo books really humanize the treatment, and also can give you and the team a quick pick me up from time to time.

Testimonial Posters Around the Office

Not all of your patients will feel comfortable becoming a poster, but some will love the idea. So, if someone's willing to mug for the camera, get a great shot, a quote about OAT, and make a poster! You can have a few frames and rotate through the sleep patients every six months or so so that your regular patients get to see different people every time they come in.

Some of my patients are shy about giving testimonials or appearing on film or in photos, but others are super enthusiastic, especially if the appliance was the first step towards having energy and being able to look and feel better. So I don't push the shy ones. And sometimes, 6 or 12 months out, a formerly shy patient is ready to speak!

Let Your Successes Speak for Themselves

If you have a patient who is super excited about their treatment at the 3, 6, or 12-month appointments (or an annual follow-up) as if they're willing to write a short note of encouragement to a new patient who is coming in for a sleep screening. Your patients remember how nerve-wracking that first appointment was, and how great it felt to finally be well-rested. So let them communicate that joy, old patient to a new patient.

Follow the Numbers

The most important thing about sleep dentistry isn't the numbers we serve, it's the life we change, but numbers can be pretty fun too. Consider putting up a sign that says something like "Thanks to Sleep Dentistry, ____ of our patients are getting a better night's sleep" and update the count every time you start a new patient on an oral appliance or PAP therapy. Over time, that number will grow, and you, your team, and your patients can take pride in that accomplishment.

Get a Photo Board

Orthodontists have boards with photos of their patients after treatment. Get a "Sleep patients served" board and put up those photos. Your patients will love finding themselves, their family, and friends, and new patients will have the comfort of knowing you've helped ordinary people, just like them. You can even give it a cute name like "Members of the Lullaby Guild" or something similar. Get a little creative and have fun! You've earned the right to brag a bit!

Choose a Sleep Patient of the Month

Pick a new sleep patient every month. Choose someone who is complying well with treatment and seeing changes in their life. Invite them in, give them balloons in a gift card, take their picture and make a little display for the front desk! Honor them on your social pages as well. Knowing that compliance gets recognition will energize your current sleep patients, and it's another 'touch point' for future sleep patients.

Keep a Memory Book of Your Favorite Patients

When you and your team feel tired and run down, look over the list of the people you've helped and the lives you've changed. You're making a huge difference for your patients, your families, and your communities. You're inspiring them to live full lives and to smile, so let their success stories inspire you! After all, they're your success stories too!

Implementation on Target!

After this chapter, you should:

- Refine your plan for getting testimonials from patients
- Set up a place in the office to celebrate sleep successes
- Plan for how you'll share your successes when they come, which will be very soon!

11: How to Handle Medical Billing

In this chapter you'll learn:

- **Basic tools to have ready to help with medical billing**
- **Key definitions for successful medical billing**
- **How the first phone call impacts billing**
- **How to verify insurance**
- **How to get the GAP exception for your patients**
- **How to get paid**
- **Why reference numbers are king**

When an office is ready to start Sleep Medicine, the biggest roadblock for the team is usually billing. Our teams can wrap their heads around taking blood pressure, treating medical issues, and saving lives. They've had to call medical providers in the past, doing it more often isn't frightening as long as their workflows are set up appropriately. Imaging and oral appliances just make sense, they're a normal part of dental office life. But medical billing? That's where we get the meltdowns.

It makes sense. We've all had to deal with our personal medical insurers when they're denying claims. We all cringe when we have to call, knowing that we'll be hours on the phone and sent through a circle of menu options. So, the thought of having to deal with that from the provider side is scary for our billing teams.

I want you to know that you can do this. My office has been successfully billing medical insurance for sleep appliances for nearly ten years. What we've found is that there are several keys to medical billing:

- Gather documentation carefully
- Make calls from a quiet, interruption-free place
- Always record the reference number given to you on a call
- File information carefully, and use color-coding to make it easier
- Expect to have to go back and forth a few times to get paid

When you do this, you're setting the stage for success.

For my office, the biggest hurdle to starting the sleep dentistry program was the billing. We hadn't done much medical billing in the past, and when we'd tried it had been grueling and frustrating. I am so glad I got my whole office team to take the class with me so that they could learn about billing in ways that made sense to them.

Tools Your Team Needs for Medical Billing

One reason our teams find medical billing difficult is that the forms, codes, and processes are different from those involved in dental billing. Our billing teams can do dental billing in their sleep. They don't have to stop and look things up, they know the forms from memory, they're used to the insurer's and their phone trees. Medical billing is hard because there's no "muscle memory" for the task. Every step takes thinking and checking and double-checking until they're familiar with the process. And that takes brainwork. (If any of your billing team members have SDB issues, maybe get them an appliance made before they have to learn this so that it's a bit easier.)

To make medical billing easier, your teams need forms that collect and organize all the information that they'll be giving and getting, checklists to help them through the steps and uninterrupted time for medical billing. If they have to switch between medical and dental all day, there's too much time lost, because they need to keep reorienting themselves to a different system. Instead, it's easier to set some blocks of time aside for medical billing and some for dental billing, keeping in mind that everything to do with medical billing takes much longer. If your office is large enough, let your billing team specialize. Choose one person to be the medical person, and let them prioritize medical billing in their daily workflow. The more your office does this, the easier it will be, but it's important to reserve time and space because medical insurance can be complicated.

If you've taken classes with me, you can find downloadable forms and checklists in my resources section. If not, take some time after this chapter to create forms and lists to support your staff, and consider getting them training in how to bill medical insurance for sleep dentistry.

The Medical Billing Workflow: Key Terms

To get started with medical billing for sleep apnea, your team will need to learn some new terms. Make a copy of this list, print it, laminate it and hang it in your billing office. Eventually, they'll be second nature, but for now, you don't want your team to have to Google every time these terms come up.

Diagnosis Code – All medical billing needs to include a diagnosis code. For sleep medicine, there is one main one that we always use: G47.33. This is the code for OSA. In the 2021 code update, there is also a code G47.8, other sleep disorders. This is the preferred code for UARS if a patient isn't severe enough for an OSA diagnosis yet.

CPT/Procedure Codes – There are 5 main procedure codes we use in the treatment of SDB. E0486 describes the oral appliance. 99203 covers the initial office visit. 70355 covers the imaging if you bill that separately. 99213 is used for follow-up visits, and 95800 is used for an HST (if permitted in your state).

DME – Durable medical equipment. This is how medical insurers cover the appliance.

Co-insurance – For some insurance, patients will have to pay co-insurance. Rather than a set copay, this is a percent split. If the insurance is 70-30, your patient will pay 30% of the cost and the insurer will pay 70. This tends to happen when an insurer bills your services as out of network.

Copay – These are set by the plan and are a fixed payment from the patient at the time of service. There's a huge variety in copay levels, and the same company will have different copays for different levels of a plan, so always check this carefully.

Pre-determination – This is an optional process where you submit all your paperwork to the insurer and they tell you if that sort of treatment is covered. It's a yes/no. They won't give you an estimate of benefits and this is not a substitute for preauthorization.

Pre-authorization – This is usually mandatory for sleep appliances, but always ASK if there is mandatory preauthorization and what it entails. To receive preauthorization, you generally need to submit all relevant medical notes and records, a statement of inability to use the CPAP, and any other supporting documentation. Pre-authorization should give you a clear statement of what the plan will cover and what the cost to the patient will be.

GAP Coverage/PPO Waver/Network Deficiency – Each insurance company has different rules for activating this clause. Basically, it means that if there is not an in-network provider for OAT within a certain radius of the patient's home, your services can be billed as in-network for one time only. This does not change your rate of pay but allows the patient to use in-network benefits and makes the appliance more affordable.

OOP Max – You're probably familiar with this from your own health insurance. Most policies have an out-of-pocket max for the year. Once this is met, the insurance covers 100% of the patient's costs.

Step 1: The New Sleep Patient Phone Call

The first point of contact for a new sleep patient is the phone call to set up an appointment. Your front desk team ***must*** take down the information important for a sleep patient (as opposed to a general or cosmetic dentistry patient). Color code your sleep patient forms and make sure that they include:

- Where the patient heard about your office (for ROI tracking)
- Details of their condition
- Address
- Employer
- Medical Insurance information including the name of the insurer, the group number, the policy number, and the phone number on the back of the card
- Any dental benefits information
- ESS screening over the phone, or direct them to the website

Remember that these sleep calls will take more time than a normal new patient call. Often these patients have arrived at your office after a journey, and they want to tell their stories. Take the time to listen, and write down any relevant info about how not sleeping is affecting their lives. This will help later with our SOAP (Subjective, Objective, Assessment, Plan) notes for the case, because it gives insight into the patient's subjective experience.

Always ask for both medical and dental insurance information. Patients often mix these up so get the information for both. You'll also need their address at this call because it will help with determining GAP coverage.

Step 2: Verifying with Insurance

The person who takes the call should record all the relevant information on the sleep patient call sheet, and then deliver that sheet to your medical billing person.

The medical billing person will copy that information from the initial call onto a form used to guide the conversation with insurance. I use these forms to make sure that every question is asked every time. Otherwise, it's easy to miss key questions, and, in general, insurers will not volunteer information. If you don't ask the right questions, it can slow down the process.

On the call, ask about:

What sleep appliance treatment is covered for your patient, what is required to get the appliance, and what the benefits are. Ask if pre-authorization is required and if GAP coverage is available given the patient's address. Find out as much about the financials as you can, and ask specifically about coverage requirements for our big 5 CPT codes: E0486, 99203, 70355, 99213, and 95800. Each policy may have different requirements, so it's important to know what documentation and supporting details you need before the first appointment.

Remember, anytime you deal with an insurer, log the call, the reference number, and the authorization number. These are very important for later when you inevitably have to contest claims.

In my team's experience, dealing with medical insurance as a provider is just as frustrating as when you're approaching them as a patient. They love rejecting claims! So be patient, expect this to take time, and buy your billing team treats. They'll need it!

Getting the GAP Exemption for Your Patients

The GAP exemption makes it easier for your patients to afford care, and that makes them more likely to say yes. This exemption causes the insurance to treat you as an in-network provider for the appliance, even though you're not in-network. Using this exemption won't make your practice permanently in-network and you don't have to change your fee structures.

What this does for the patient:

- Your services will count towards their in-network (usually lower) deductible
- Their co-insurance rate will be lower
- You will count towards their (lower) in-network OOP maximum

- Some plans only HAVE in-network benefits, this lets the patient use them

Basically, it makes the appliance a better bargain for them, especially if they're close to their deductible for the year. If GAP is denied, you'll just be treated as an out-of-network provider, so it's important to have both cost estimates ready for the patient. You can phrase it as "Your out-of-network cost will be *x*, but if we can get the GAP exemption, we can save you some money."

Some insurance firms allow you to file for the GAP exemption. In other cases, the patient has to call and start the process.

Get to Know Your Insurer Websites

More and more, insurers are improving their websites so that you can get estimates of benefits, GAP coverage, and even preauthorization using secure online document portals instead of faxes. This saves time, money, and headaches for your team.

Step 3: Getting Paid

Now we get to the fun part – the part where insurers pay you for your services! Actually, it's not much fun. But if you and the team stay calm and keep all those reference numbers handy, you'll be able to make it through the process.

First of all, you may have to resubmit the clinical issue. Yes, you've already submitted this two or three times, but they'll ask for it again. Include the signed delivery form from appliance delivery. Make sure you completed the work within the authorized date range, and submit all approvals. If you're not filing the claim online, use a CMS 1500 form.

Most GAP claims will be processed out of network on the first try, and many pre-authorized claims will also be rejected.

This does not mean that you messed up. Medical insurers often make mistakes in processing claims. (You probably have experience with this from your personal life.) Make sure that you warn patients that they may get a notice from the insurer that the claim is rejected, but not to worry, you'll handle it.

Check each claim report received against what you expected to be paid and how you expected it to work with the patient's plan. Call the insurer to contest the claim, and use the reference numbers from earlier conversations. This will usually get them to reprocess. Record the reference number from this call too!

Sometimes, we'll have to ask for the same claim to be reprocessed 2 or 3 times before the insurer finally gets it right. The key is to be persistent and document every single contact you have with the insurance company, from the first confirmation of benefits call onward.

Billing medical insurance is a big change from billing dental insurance, so you may want to get your team training in this. However, if everyone keeps trying and is detail-oriented about documentation, it will soon seem almost as easy as dental.

Implementation on Target!

After this chapter you should:

- Download or create forms to help your team navigate new patient sleep calls and medical insurance calls
- Choose a team member to be the point person for medical billing
- Get that person training, either by teaching them yourself or sending them to class
- Learn the terms for medical billing so you can answer questions
- Find ways to remind the team: Reference number, reference number, reference number
- Set up medical provider accounts with the major insurers

12: Getting Started Seeing Patients

Now it's time to get into the details of implementation. Right now, you probably have a few big questions:

How will a sleep patient move through the office?

How much time do my team and I need to reserve for sleep patients?

How will I collect the documentation for the case?

How will I conduct the examination? What tools do I need to have on hand?

How will I score sleep questionnaires and discuss them with patients?

Do I need a script, or can I adlib?

How will my team participate in the process?

What can we do to smooth transitions?

Am I actually able to identify OSA patients with my current skill set?

I can't answer these questions for you, because every team and practice is different. To find answers to these questions, you'll need to jump in and start working with patients.

Your First Sleep Appointments

Your first sleep patients can be team members, or family and friends. You want them to be willing to help you iron out bugs in your new systems, and honest enough to tell you what's working, what's not, and what can be tweaked a little.

I went into this assuming that my appointments would have to be a lot longer to incorporate sleep screenings, and I was surprised. We ended up eliminating some of the "dead time" in appointments, where patients were sitting and waiting. The actual appointments weren't much longer, and to the patients, they felt shorter!

Checklist for a Successful Practice Sleep Dentistry Appointment

As you hone your skills on your volunteers, you'll want to follow a checklist so that you don't miss any key steps. You can create your own list. However, make sure it includes, at the bare minimum, the following items:

- Insurance check and confirmation of benefits before the appointment
- Screening questionnaire
- Complete health history
- Explanation of why you're conducting a sleep screening and the problems poor sleep causes
- Weight and height
- Blood pressure
- Neck circumference
- Observation of breathing
- Physical examination of molars, tongue, palate, tonsils, and throat
- Discussion of screening and exam results
- If necessary, education on the next steps for UARS or OSA, and treatment options for these conditions
- Information on referrals
- Education on OAT and why it can help
- "Healthy sleep" gift bag with information and some branded item (like a sleep mask)

Which Screening Questions Should I Use?

Different sleep screening tools identify different subgroups of sleep patients.

Everyone I talked to has the same story. We decided to add sleep dentistry to our practices. While learning our way around the screening tools, we administered them to ourselves and our loved ones. And, we found SDB where we hadn't expected it! The first lives we saved were our own lives and the lives of the people closest to us. These screening tools are so simple to use, and they change lives.

STOP-BANG – screening tool is simple to administer and, except for neck size and BMI, is simply a series of yes or no questions. It's excellent at picking up people with moderate to severe OSA, so it's a good first-line questionnaire.

ESS – The Epworth Sleepiness scale is useful for identifying people who may not be overweight, but who aren't getting good rest. The scale assesses self-reported daytime sleepiness by having the patient identify situations where they're likely to doze off.

PSQI – Pittsburgh Sleep Quality Index is more thorough than the ESS. The benefit is that it is very good at catching UARS before it progresses to full-blown OSA, even in cases where the patient is not experiencing excessive daytime sleepiness. The drawback is that this evaluation takes longer for the patient to take and the team to score.

Most practices should choose at least 2 screenings for their patients to help the greatest number of people. Initially, you may want to administer different combinations of the three screening tools. Find out which one hits your ideal spot in terms of identifying patients with problems without being too complicated for the patients or team to complete and score.

If the Patient is Providing a Health History, Why do we Also Need to Check Height, Weight, Blood Pressure, and Neck Size?

You'll ask each sleep patient to provide a complete health history. However, many of your regular patients may have not had a routine physical recently. Or, when they're filling out forms, they may rush and forget key info. Taking a few objective measurements can give you important information your patients may have forgotten.

Height and weight let you compute an accurate BMI

Large necks are an important risk factor for OSA

Blood pressure is important to spot hypertension. Many people never check their blood pressure and don't realize that there's a problem until they're already in crisis. This is why hypertension is known as the "silent killer."

If your patients ask about all the "medical stuff" as part of a dental appointment, explain that there is a link between sleep, oral health, and whole-body health and that these physical signs can help identify patients with UARS and OSA.

What Should I Look For as I Observe a Patient's Breathing?

Often, by the time the screening tools are complete, the breathing exam and the physical exam are almost superfluous. However, it can be important for determining underlying causes for OSA or for catching UARS patients who might otherwise slip under the radar. During this part of the exam, be especially alert for:

- Mouth breathing
- Nose noises like whistling or snorting
- Irregular breathing patterns that indicate a struggle to breathe

What Should I Look for During the Physical Exam?

- A high, narrow palate
- An unrevised tongue-tie. Have them demonstrate their tongue's range of movement to ensure that they can easily reach the roof of the mouth
- A fatty tongue, which could block the airway
- A floppy, poorly toned soft palate
- Signs of tooth grinding or clenching
- Enlarged tonsils – while these are more common in children, adults with sleep breathing issues may have inflamed tonsils as well

Make note of any irregularities in the patient's chart.

What Should I Do Besides Examining and Educating?

During your first sleep appointments, time yourself and your patient. You'll want to examine the process and decide which parts should be delegated.

- How long does it take your patients to fill out the screening questionnaires?
- Would it be better to have an electronic form the patients can complete before they arrive at the office?
- How long does it take you to check height, weight, BP, and neck circumference?
- Are these tasks that would be better delegated to a dental assistant, or do you prefer to do them yourself?
- How long does the oral sleep apnea exam take?
- Can you quickly identify abnormalities?
- How can you incorporate this into a normal exam?
- How long does it take to answer questions?
- Do your patients have a lot of questions?
- How long does a referral take?
- Do you have prewritten referral forms?

- Will you have your office team assist in setting up appointments with specialists, or will you leave that to the patient?
- Can you and your team quickly complete the imaging/scans or impressions for an oral appliance?
- How quickly can your patients get a sleep study or ENT appointment?

These first patients will help you perfect your systems and processes so that your sleep program meshes with the existing office schedule, get patients seen and tested quickly, and provides clear options in a known time frame.

What Should I Do After the Sleep Appointment?

Ensure that any referrals for patients who presented with sleep issues are completed. Follow up and see where the patients are having trouble moving ahead. Are they having to wait too long to see the physicians you refer them to? Is it too hard to book a sleep study? Keep track of which patients return to you for additional treatment, such as an oral appliance.

Send each of your early patients a thank you note. Include referral cards, in case they have family or friends to refer for a sleep screening.

Sit down with key team members, review how long each part of the appointment took, and develop a plan for streamlining the process and delegating tasks. This is a new program. You're still refining your systems. If you encounter problems, it means that your system isn't done!

What are Some Systems That Have Worked for Other Offices?

Many offices start out slowly, doing only one or two sleep appointments a day. If you do this, it gives you a chance to perfect your part of the sleep appointments and to teach your team to handle their roles. Once you understand the flow and the timing, you can add more sleep appointments into your schedule.

Not all office flows are going to look the same. For instance, here are two different ways of running a sleep appointment.

Workflow A: Small Office, Minimal Space

When the patient makes the appointment, the team collects medical and dental insurance information. Medical benefits for sleep medicine are confirmed before the first appointment. At this time the team can put together a patient-specific referral list that works with their insurance.

The patient arrives at the office and checks in.

The front desk completes the check-in process and hands patient screening forms with instructions to fill them out as much as possible.

The patient turns in the forms and is escorted back to the chair

The front desk scores forms using a scoring guide.

The hygiene appointment begins. Before starting the cleaning, a hygienist measures and records weight, height, neck circumference, and blood pressure.

During the hygiene appointment, the front office gives screening results to the dentist. The hygienist records any signs of sleep apnea for the dentist to confirm.

Dental examination. In addition to the annual oral cancer screening, the dentist checks the mouth for signs and causes of sleep apnea. She talks about what she is looking for and why.

Sleep education. After the examination, the dentist discusses the patient's UARS and OSA risk factors. If the patient is at risk, she explains how diagnosis and treatment can help and asks if the patient would like a referral.

If the patient wants a referral, the desk team calls and sets up the appointment for him.

After the sleep study has been completed, the dental office can follow up with treatment options and set up a treatment appointment.

Workflow B: Larger Office, Bigger Team

When the patient makes the appointment, the team collects medical and dental insurance information. Medical benefits for sleep medicine are confirmed before the first appointment.

The patient arrives and completes the normal check-in process.

The Dental Assistant escorts the patient to the room then performs height, weight, neck size, and BP screens. DA educates briefly about why the office now offers sleep dentistry and why sleep is important.

The DA administers screenings to the patient and makes note of any additional info that comes out during the screening. DA gives a small amount of education.

The hygienist begins cleaning while the DA goes over the sleep screen results with the Dentist.

Dental exam. The dentist mentions the patient's risk factors for UARS and OSA based on screening. Makes note of any underlying issues with the palate, tongue, jaw, or tonsils.

The dentist offers an opinion on whether the patient should seek a sleep study, explains treatment options, and why the sleep study is necessary (So that insurance will cover PAP or OAT.).

The benefits coordinator presents referrals, insurance info, and estimated cost.

After DX is confirmed, the office calls the patient to schedule a follow-up appointment for treatment.

You don't need a big team to start with dental sleep medicine. When I started, I only had three team members! The key to success is making sure everyone knows what their role is, and ensuring that the processes mean that no team member is overwhelmed or falling behind. As your program grows, keep an eye out for opportunities to grow your team as well!

My first few sleep appointments were so clumsy and disorganized! I felt terrible and was ready to give up, but I reminded myself that this was important work for my patients. I sat down with the team, and we analyzed what was going wrong, why, and how to fix it. Having a good system and clear expectations for every step made a huge difference!

Roadblocks to Implementation

Here are a few common roadblocks my students have encountered, and advice on how to address them in your practice.

Road Block # 1 The Screenings are too Long

If you administer all 3 screenings on paper, it's a lot of work for the patient. Some patients are faster at forms than others, some get fatigued, and some get annoyed. Then, someone in the office has to score all those screenings while the appointment is going on. The easiest way around this roadblock is to have a DA administer the screenings in the following order:

Weight, Height, Neck Size, and BP

STOP-BANG

ESS

PSQI

This order allows you to minimize the number of screenings. If STOP-BANG shows that a patient is at risk and needs a sleep study, you can skip the other screenings. If ESS shows a risk, you can skip PSQI. You only need to use PSQI for patients who passed the other screenings. This will cut down on time and patient inconvenience.

It's also more pleasant for most patients to talk their way through a screening than to fill out a huge number of forms.

Road Block #2 - The Physicians and Sleep Labs we Have Relationships With Aren't in Every Patient's Network

First of all, as a dentist, you're never going to be in-network. In some cases, patients are just going to have to pay for out-of-network care if they want their sleep issues addressed.

Give your patients the best estimate of the cost that you can, and let them decide if their health is worth the cost when their insurance won't pay.

Road Block #3 - Sleep Screening Adds too Much Time to My Appointments

This can be an issue, especially if you start running behind and leaving patients waiting. Going forward, you'll want to block appointments differently to leave more time for screening. There are a few ways to do this.

You can have longer new patient and "once a year screening" appointment blocks. You can reserve certain days for sleep dentistry, certain days for Invisalign, certain days for cosmetic procedures.

You can keep your current blocks, but leave more lag in the schedule for patients who take longer to screen and educate.

You can delegate some of the education to non-clinical team members, and have it happen in a meeting area instead of a chair, to free up chair time.

How you're going to fit this service in depends on the team you have, the space you have, and the time you have. If you're unsure which option will work best, run a few more beta tests, using different models each time. Again, there's no one right way to do this. Every practice is unique, and you need to find out what is best for you and your team.

Road Block #4 - None of my Early Patients Have Shown any Signs of OSA or UARS

About 10% of Americans have SDB, and this rises to nearly 40% of Americans over 65. Most people with SDB have not been diagnosed and aren't receiving treatment. If none of your first patients had symptoms or failed their screenings, congratulations – you picked a very healthy group of family and friends. Run another test, but this time try to include more people who are older, overweight, or have high blood pressure. If you're still not identifying anyone who needs a sleep study, you may need to practice your own screening and identification skills.

After you've seen your first patients, you've completed a "Soft Launch" of your new service. Now it's time to plan for a "Hard Launch" where you announce it to patients, call local media, and spread the word about dental sleep medicine in your community!

Implementation on Target!

After this chapter, you should:

- Reach out to the people you want to be your first patients
- Conduct your first sleep appointments
- Follow up to make sure the referrals are going through and resulting in appointments.
- Analyze the appointment process and perfect your workflows
- Pick a date and plan the "Hard Launch" of your program.

Part 3: Implementing Pediatric Sleep Dentistry

Do you want to change lives, help kids grow up healthy and happy, and heal families? Then it's time to implement a pediatric sleep dentistry program in your practice.

When kids can't sleep, their schoolwork suffers, their moods suffer, their health suffers and their behavior suffers. This all adds up to suffering families. A good pediatric sleep program helps get these kids on track for healthy, successful lives, and relieves the incredible amount of stress on their parents. Remember, often these parents have looked EVERYWHERE for help for their kids. They're exhausted and they've lost hope.

On top of that, so many of the physical issues that cause pediatric sleep issues run in families. So you'll see a child with a tongue tie and a high narrow palate and poor sleep quality, and then the parents will realize that they also have the same problems. They'll have stories of needing multiple adult teeth extracted, years of speech therapy, continual nasal and sinus issues, and snoring and gagging during sleep. No professional ever linked all of these issues together, and because they "run in the family" the parents will never have realized that they're preventable and treatable.

When you implement pediatric sleep dentistry well, you change lives, you get a constant flow of adult and pediatric sleep patients, and you revitalize your practice.

So, let's get started on creating the perfect pediatric sleep program for your practice, so you can make great changes in your life and your community!

13: Identifying Your First Patients: The Power of Moms

In this chapter you'll learn:

- Why pediatric sleep dentistry is a self-marketing service
- How to bring up behavioral symptoms gently
- Why you should make sure every child has been screened for tongue and lip ties as well as palate issues

Initially, I was just looking for some CE credit. So much of the CE opportunities focuses on adults, and I wanted something for my pediatric patients. Sleep dentistry sounded interesting. I didn't really expect to add it to my own practice, I was just trying to learn something new.

The first questions a practice owner asks about expanding a service line are usually "How do I know that there's a demand for this service in my community?" and "How will I find patients who want this service?" For pediatric sleep dentistry, you can look around the community and see the signs of kids who aren't sleeping well. You can hear it in the stories of teachers, whose classrooms seem to be getting harder and harder to manage. You'll see demand as you sit at soccer or baseball practice with your own kids, and other mothers mention that they've tried and tried, but there just don't seem to be solutions for their kids.

If you have a child who needs speech therapy or occupational therapy, you can also see the demand for these services when you talk to their own therapists. Everywhere, there are kids who are mouth-breathers, who are too sleepy or too hyperactive, who wet the bed, and who have the constellation of issues that tells us that, yes, this is a kid who may need a sleep screening and who may have structural issues that cause their inability to breathe in their sleep. The need is there, and it's probably greater in your community than it has been in decades.

Why Children's Sleep Breathing is Getting Worse – Less Sleep Overall

One huge reason for the increase in children's sleep breathing problems is that children are getting less sleep overall. American sleep times have declined across all ages since the 1940s but hit rock bottom with the invention of home internet and accessible Wi-Fi.

Kids aren't sleeping because we keep them busy all day with school, sports, activities, and homework, and then put them to bed with screens to help them unwind. Instead, they stay up playing or watching Youtube videos.

If a child has sleep breathing issues but sleeps longer, they might do all right. They're not living their best life, but maybe they're still managing to get enough sleep if they stay in bed long enough or take naps every day. When a child is already sleep-deprived, as modern children are, and you add sleep breathing issues to the mix, what you get is a disaster.

Why Children's Sleep Breathing is Getting Worse – Palatal Issues

One reason that we're seeing an increase of children with sleep issues is that it is no longer standard practice to evaluate for and release tongue ties in newborns. Pediatricians are very focused on eating and growing. If a child is growing adequately, they'll often say that a tongue tie isn't important and leave it in place.

The problem is that the tongue affects more than the ability to nurse or take a bottle. An untethered tongue can rest in the palate. It acts as a natural palatal expander throughout infancy and the toddler years, especially during sleep. As the palate widens, the nasal cavity grows larger, and breathing becomes easier, even when a child has a cold or allergies.

Resting the tongue in the palate also keeps the airway open during sleep and promotes nasal breathing. A child who can't rest her tongue in her palate is going to have a restricted airway. She may snore or be prone to mouth breathing. And if anything affects her nose, like a cold or allergies, it's going to have a huge impact on her sleep breathing.

Pediatricians tend to leave palates to the dentists, so they're not worried about the effects of a tethered tongue on the development of the palate. But many children don't see a dentist until they're in preschool or kindergarten. That means they've had years of poor palate development, effects on speech (if you can't move your tongue, you can't make certain sounds), and trouble with food. These are kids who can't move food around their mouths. They choke and gag a lot. They may avoid hard-to-eat foods. And they often have sleep breathing issues going unnoticed because of their other, more obvious, problems.

I was shocked by how much the description of symptoms and breathing issues matched my own kid. And, this is embarrassing, but when her pediatrician said there was no need to clip her tongue tie, I'd gone along with it. I was a new mom, awash in hormones, and I didn't want to cause my baby unnecessary pain. I should have known better! I see tweens with palate issues in my office all the time and talk about what we can do for the kids, but when it was my own daughter? I lived with her and saw her every day, and never really thought about what the unrevised tongue tie was doing to her development.

How Families Finally Get Help

Very few dentists, even pediatric dentists, routinely screen for tongue tie and palatal issues. In fact, depending on the family's choice of orthodontist, a kid might have healthy adult teeth removed rather than get treatment for palate issues. Families are eager for solutions but don't know which providers will screen for and revise tongue and lip ties in older kids. Often, the only provider is hours away, with a huge waiting list. So, when a local dentist starts a sleep program that also addresses tongue and palate issues, moms talk to moms, and the word spreads quickly.

One mom gets help for her child. Then, at a soccer game or school event, she meets someone else who mentions similar problems. She refers them to the dentist who helped her child, and the cycle continues. Once someone in your community is providing these screenings and services, families line up for help.

This is why my implementation plan for dental offices does not include a marketing piece.

You can certainly market your new pediatric sleep program if you enjoy marketing. You should make a place for it on your website and incorporate pediatric sleep dentistry into your social media calendar, but you don't need to do a huge advertising push. This service is needed, your patients will come to you once you start screening and treating your current patients.

Your First Patients

As you launch your program, talk to the parents. While the child is in the chair, ask how they're doing in school, how they sleep, if they have any problems with attention or concentration. Find out how they're eating. Do they eat a wide variety of things, or are they picky? The reason you want to have this conversation is so that if you find evidence of breathing, tongue, or palate issues, you can connect those to the child's behavior. You want to help the parents see that this isn't just a matter of "might need braces some day" or "needs more speech therapy," but an underlying, medical cause for many of the issues their children have.

After the seminar, the first thing I did was get my daughter a sleep study. Sure enough, she had sleep breathing issues, and her tongue and palate were contributing factors. After treatment, she was a different child. School got better, home got better, her moods were better. Now, when I talk to patients about sleep apnea, high palates, and tongue tie, I don't just do it as a doctor. I can talk to them as a mom who's been where they are, and who was able to help her child.

As you check the child's tongue mobility and palate, don't just ask them to stick out their tongue. Check and see if their tongue can comfortably rest in the palate and move around the roof of the mouth. Many of your patients may never have had a thorough exam of tongue and palate because they're not quite far enough behind in any one way to trigger a clinical evaluation.

The more children that you help, the more families there are who will beat a path to your door. These kids are out there, they need help. Curing sleep breathing issues and getting kids a fresh start is the best marketing you have.

Implementation on Target!

After this chapter you should:

- Be ready to approach parents as another parent
- Start screening your pediatric patients
- Ask every parent about school, behavior, and sleep during the exam
- Check every pediatric patient for tongue tie, lip tie, and palate issues at least onc

14: Reaching Out for Referrals: Don't Forget OTs and SLPs

In this chapter you'll learn:

- Which specialists to build relationships with
- Where to find those specialists
- How to persuade them to work with your practice
- How to keep those referrals coming in

No one can run a successful pediatric sleep dentistry practice alone. You'll need the help of other professionals to diagnose your pediatric patients, to get them appropriate treatment, and to document the cases.

When I started implementing sleep dentistry, one of the parts I found most intimidating was reaching out to other specialists. I'm used to being in a bit of a solo – my patients mention their primary care physician on their forms, but unless I'm clearing them for surgery, I rarely contact them. Making these connections really forced me to step outside of my comfort zone.

Essential Specialists for Your Pediatric Sleep Program

Let's take a look at some of the specialists you'll need to build relationships with as you implement your program.

Pediatricians

Your local pediatricians can be a great resource. Many don't think in terms of tongue tie or palates unless they're dealing with a failure-to-thrive infant or a child with an identifiable genetic syndrome. They're busy and tend to think of palates as a dental issue. However, once they're educated on the relationship between tongue, palate, and sleep breathing, they can be reliable allies.

Pediatricians are also able to order sleep studies and examine tonsils and adenoids (though it's often easier to get a good look at tonsils in the dental chair.) They're an especially important resource if you practice in an area without a pediatric ENT within a reasonable drive. While some parents may have the time to drive their child an hour or more each way to a specialist's appointment, other families might forego care if you refer to a physician who is too far away. Pediatricians can be important for bridging those gaps in accessible care.

ENT

To operate a successful pediatric sleep dentistry program, it's important to have an ENT who you can refer children with enlarged tonsils and adenoids to, especially since a tonsillectomy and adenoidectomy is the first line of treatment for pediatric OSA in the absence of other underlying physical conditions. A good ENT can also help kids whose blockage is a combination of a high, narrow palate and environmental allergies. You have the tools to appropriately treat the underlying physical problems, the ENT can treat the nasal and lung issues, and together, you can resolve the sleep breathing problems.

Allergist

You'll find that many of your pediatric sleep patients also suffer from untreated or undertreated allergies, with dust and mold being some of the biggest culprits. For the best outcomes, it's important to get those allergies addressed. Kids who are fussy eaters can also benefit from an appointment. Sometimes, kids have a limited diet because their tongue and palate make it hard to move food around their mouths, or because the stress of not sleeping makes it harder for them to eat, but sometimes an underlying food allergy is driving both food preferences and their ability to sleep.

Gastroenterologist

If you don't already have a relationship with a GI, get one. Many children with OSA also have acid reflux. Mouth breathing a tongue-tie can also cause stomach pain and other issues. And GI issues can also interfere with sleep and cause frequent waking. If you're serious about solving these issues, it can help to have a GI on call.

Cardiologist

Why would a child without congenital defects need to see a cardiologist? Well, if they have OSA, they may already have high blood pressure or cardiovascular damage. As the pediatric OSA epidemic gets worse, more and more kids are showing up with high blood pressure and heart damage at younger ages. A relationship with a cardiologist means that you have somewhere to refer these kids and that they have someone to work with when kids aren't cured by surgery and can't tolerate the PAP machine, or whose issues are caused by the tongue and the palate.

Endocrinologist

Kids with OSA are also at higher risk for Type II Diabetes and may have growth problems (since the body needs sleep to grow.) While most patients you see, won't need an endocrinologist, it's worth having a good one to recommend.

Pediatric Sleep Lab

It's important to know which sleep labs in your area do pediatric sleep studies and to have their contact information available to patients. However, with pediatric patients, your first referral will usually be to an ENT since the standard, first-line treatment for pediatric OSA is typically a T&A.

Local Occupational Therapists

There are two reasons to build a relationship with local occupational therapists. First of all, after you release ties and expand palates, some children may need extra help learning how to breathe, chew and swallow. A good OT can help a child with these muscle tasks. Children who have suffered from OSA for a long time may also benefit from social and behavioral interventions since they were too tired to learn these skills when all their age-mates learned them.

The other reason it's important to let your local OTs know what you're doing is that they see a lot of children who may have underlying sleep, tongue, or palate issues. They need someone to refer those patients to, and in many communities, you may be the only dentist who has an active pediatric sleep program. Building connections is a two-way street. Everyone wants to help these kids, but not everyone has built a strong team yet. You can be the person who pulls the team together.

Local Speech and Language Pathologists

Sleep and Language Pathologists (SLPs) are another natural ally. Did you know that the failure to revise tongue and lip ties at birth lands many children in speech therapy later in life? SLPs understand the importance of breathing and how palates and tongues affect sleep and breathing. They're good at documenting how sleep issues and structural issues are causing problems for a child. Often, the big problem is that there's no one local practicing pediatric sleep dentistry. Their patients need help and there's no one to refer them to.

On the flipside, your sleep apnea kids may also need SLP services. The school SLPs are overworked in most areas, but parents may not know where to find a private SLP with time to see their child. By working together, you can get these kids sleeping right, breathing right, and ready to grow.

How to Reach Out to Specialists

I decided to start with the easiest ones – my children's own physicians and speech therapists. I was surprised at how enthusiastic the reception was. There are so many kids who weren't cured after T&A, who can't tolerate the CPAP, and who need help. Other specialists just weren't sure if anyone locally was doing this kind of medicine! Once I had the confidence from approaching people I knew, I was ready to approach strangers.

The most important thing to know when reaching out to pediatric specialists is that your services are in demand and you are serving a real need. For instance, the website UpToDate.com discusses the benefits of pediatric sleep dentistry for children with OSA (https://www.uptodate.com/contents/management-of-obstructive-sleep-apnea-in-children). Often, appliances can cure or greatly improve apnea Hypopnea indices without surgery, and in severe cases, surgery and an appliance can achieve greater results than surgery alone.

So why aren't more children receiving these services? According to the site, it's because, "If the clinician and patient choose to pursue this therapy, the first step is an evaluation by a trained sleep dentist with certification in dental sleep medicine to evaluate the child's oral cavity and potential tolerance to the device. ***This specialized expertise is important and may not be available in many areas*** (emphasis added)" You're a pediatric sleep dentist now, and you can help these kids.

Remember, however, that specialists are just as busy as you are. What do you do when you get a letter about some new program or service? Do you act on it right away? Or does it take multiple touches before you're interested? While specialists who know you personally may be immediately enthusiastic about your new program, other members of the local medical community may need more time and encouragement. To engage them, you're going to need to make multiple contacts in multiple ways.

If you've already read the adult section on getting referrals, you'll notice some similarities to the earlier section. However, there will be some differences since, unless you practice near a major children's hospital, pediatric specialists may be harder to find than adult specialists.

Finding Specialists Step 1: Making the Lists

So, how will you decide which physicians and specialists you'll contact about your pediatric sleep dentistry program? The first step is to find out which practices in your area see pediatric patients or are affiliated with regional children's hospitals and host pediatric specialists for clinics a few times a month.

Start by calling local pediatricians and family practice doctors, and see who they make referrals to. Then research the children's hospitals that cover your area, and see if they come to town for clinics.

Once you have a list of pediatric specialists, it's time to let them know what you're doing, why you're doing it, and why you want a working relationship with them.

Step 2: Focus on Developing Educational Programs

A great way to add to your list of potential specialists and to increase interest in your sleep dentistry program is to offer educational programming. Are there study groups for physicians and specialists in your area, either independently or through a hospital system? Volunteer to offer a program and provide food.

Most physicians only receive a brief introduction to sleep medicine in medical school or their residencies. Many have no idea of how sleep disturbances present in pediatric patients, or how a pediatric sleep dentist can help open airways so that children can breathe better. So, get out there and educate your local medical community! Bring notepads or business cards with your office information along. Remember, pediatric sleep dentists are fairly rare. Many physicians in the community haven't recommended patients for this treatment because no one was providing it!

The materials from your educational programs will also be handy as you reach out to specialists. You'll already have the words and information you need to make a convincing "pitch" for your sleep services.

Step 3: Making Contact

The next step is to reach out to the people on your list. Keep in mind that you may have to contact them more than once before you get a response. Start with a letter explaining what your new sleep program will entail, why you're contacting them, and how to get in touch with you to discuss options. You can also include a form for them to return if they'd like to be part of a mutual referral program.

Your letter may look something like this. Feel free to take this general format and customize it for your own practice and specialists.

February 2, 2022

Dear Dr. Jones,

I am a local dentist who is adding pediatric sleep dentistry to my practice. Sleep dentistry identifies and treats patients with Sleep Disordered Breathing in a dental practice setting through the use of appliances that correct palatal issues, improve tongue positioning, and help develop and keep the airway open during sleep.

As part of treating the underlying issues contributing to my patients' sleep breathing issues, I would like to be able to refer them to a <insert specialty>. May I refer patients in need of <specialty> services to your office for care?

While I am adding this service to benefit my existing patients, I am also able to take referrals for non-patients who have palate or tongue issues affecting their sleep breathing. For many children, a combination of surgery and an oral appliance are needed to reduce the apnea hypopnea index (AHI) and restore healthy sleep.

I am passionate about getting as many children as possible help for their sleep breathing problems, and therapy is only effective if patients can comply with it. Please let me know if your office can help my patients by accepting referrals for diagnosis.

Sincerely,

<name>

After you send the letter, follow up. Even if a physician is willing to partner with your pediatric sleep program, they may set the letter aside, intending to respond later. About 14 days after you mail the letters, you should follow up with a phone call. In most cases, you'll talk to the office manager, not the physician. In the call you should:

- Ask the letter was received
- Ask if the physician has any questions
- Ask if there is a specific fax, phone, or email to use when referring patients
- Offer to send another letter
- Leave your contact information

Step 4: Choose a Team Member to Work on These Relationships

Good relationships take work. It's a cliché from self-help books, but it also applies to your relationships with pediatric specialists. If the clinical side of the practice keeps you too busy to maintain relationships with the physicians who you refer to and who refer to you, then a team member needs to step up.

One way to manage these relationships is with a simple spreadsheet or table, tracking name, specialty, contact info, and what contacts have been made, and on which dates.

Keep track of how many referrals go back and forth between your practices, what your last contact with each office was, and when you should get back in touch with them. Examples of contacts are:

- Updates on patients
- Thank you notes for referrals or for helping a patient get diagnosed
- Newsletters
- Small tokens of appreciation
- Calls
- Visits to their office by you or a team member
- Emails
- Meetings at luncheons or other professional events
- Direct mailers
- Facebook and LinkedIn connections
- Local professional groups online and in-person

The more personalized your contacts can be, the better. You want these other practitioners to remember that you exist, that you appreciate their help with your patients, and that you provide great care to their patients. Frequent contacts mean that when they have a patient who couldn't get or didn't see improvement with a T&A, can't tolerate PAP therapy, or who has underlying teeth, tongue, or palate issues, they'll think of you.

To keep up with these relationships, choose a team member who is outgoing, cheerful, and intelligent. If their current duties won't give them time to help build your referral program, it's time to change up job descriptions and redistribute workloads. Building a good 2-way referral network is essential for practicing sleep dentistry.

Step 5: Making Your First Sleep Dentistry Referrals

Once you've begun to make contact with the specialists in your areas, you can make your first sleep dentistry referrals. These might be for the children of family, office team members, and friends, or they may be for patients. Eventually, you'll develop bidirectional relationships with these specialists, but for now, it's up to you to take the first step.

For pediatric patients, most of your referrals will be to ENTs. That's because, in the absence of obvious tongue and palate issues, the first line of treatment for a child with OSA is a T&A, and the ENT will be the one to determine if they need a sleep study and surgery. Even children who need tongue-tie revision and a palatal expander should see the ENT to help with documenting the medical need for these procedures.

The second most common referral you'll make is to the allergist. That's because many children with sleep breathing problems also have allergy and asthma issues. You'll get the best results if you can correct physical problems restricting the airway while at the same time reducing or eliminating swelling or irritation from allergies.

Remember, in children, sleep-disordered breathing is often caused by several factors acting together. Correcting one of them helps a little, but correcting all of the contributing issues will make a huge difference in the child's life and health.

If you are having trouble finding pediatric ENTs, you may want to first refer the child to her own pediatrician. This is also important when the insurer wants all referrals to come from the PCP. It's important to clarify rules and benefits before you make referrals so that you can get the child connected with care as quickly as possible.

When you make the referral, first talk to the parents. Explain that you're seeing signs of SDB, but you need to refer to an ENT so that the child can receive a medical diagnosis and have treatment covered by health insurance. Reassure them that the ENT is a good doctor, great with kids, and ready to help.

Have your office team call in the referral and set up an appointment for your patient. It's important to complete this step before the patient leaves the office. Otherwise, the parents may intend to set up an appointment later, but never get around to it.

Check with the parents after the appointment to see how it went, and follow up with the doctor that you referred them to. Were they sent for a sleep study? Why or why not? If they were not sent for a sleep study, what documentation does the doctor need to order one? Some specialists are more conservative about diagnosing sleep-disordered breathing than others. If the ENT sends a child back when you can clearly see sleep problems, you can write up a letter explaining the issues you've seen and that the teachers and parents have seen, and ask them to reconsider the data. Because the first-line treatment for kids is surgery, some ENTs prefer to take a "wait and see" approach.

If you find that you are referring to a specialist who doesn't take your observations or your patients' experiences seriously, stop. Find a new specialist who is willing to diagnose UARS and mild OSA so that your patients can get help before their disease progresses to weight gain, high blood pressure, or diabetes.

Step 6: Make Sure You Follow Up

Follow up with the parents and the specialist to find out when the sleep study occurred and what the results are. If the child was borderline for OSA or UARS, remember that symptoms matter. If someone is subclinical on a sleep study but falls asleep in class or is a danger to other students, it's a medical emergency and deserves immediate treatment.

If you need to pull together extra documentation for insurance, now is the time. The Epworth Sleepiness Scale can be a big help here. So can evidence from teachers and coaches, and also any growth or biomarker issues. Resubmit your evidence to the specialist, and keep pushing for a diagnosis. Your patient needs help, or they're running the risk of short-term death from accidents and long-term injury from cardiovascular disease, obesity, and diabetes.

Step 7: Send a Thank You

After you've gotten a patient a diagnosis, send a thank you note to the specialist who diagnosed them with UARS or OSA. Highlight how they've improved the patient's life, and mention that you hope to work with them in the future. Thanking specialists serves two purposes. It expresses your appreciation so that they'll diagnose your future referrals, and it keeps your practice in their memory so that they'll choose you for their oral appliance patients. Remember, your goal for any of these professional relationships is a two-way referral stream.

Why Add Professionals Who Can't Diagnose to Your Referral Network?

It's important to also build connections with non-physicians like occupational therapists, sleep and language pathologists, and Myofunctional therapists. Why? Because getting your patients the therapy they need can improve their success with sleep apnea treatment, and because many of these professionals see many children who have tongue and palate issues, are habitual mouth breathers, and who show signs of sleep-disordered breathing. When dentists and therapists focused on oral-motor issues work together, everyone's patients see better outcomes.

Building relationships with these professionals works much like building them with physicians. Outreach, education, and being friendly and approachable will help you build connections that get your patients and their patients the help that they need.

I hit my first roadblock with the ENT. The first one I tried told everyone they'd grow out of it. He wouldn't even order sleep studies for the kids with tongue ties and high palates! The hands-off approach wasn't getting these kids help, and meanwhile, they were falling behind in school and life. I had to approach a second ENT, who was farther away but who was more educated about sleep issues. So, I'd urge you to keep trying. If one specialist won't work with you, find one who will. Pediatric sleep medicine is still an emerging field, and many specialists don't have time to stay up to date on the latest developments.

Roadblocks to Building Your Referral Network

A good relationship with area physicians is the first step to a successful sleep practice. So, what do you do when you're not getting anywhere? Why isn't anyone responding to your calls and emails? Why do your team members report that reaching out in person doesn't work? If you're hitting a roadblock on building a referral network, here are some hints that can help you out.

If You're in a Smaller Town or Suburb

If you're in a smaller town or suburb, you may face issues because pediatric specialists don't practice in your town. Instead, they're part of larger networks and may already have their own preferred dental providers.

In this case, try reaching out to your local PCPs instead. Maybe you need to connect with nurse practitioners if they're the group providing most of the day-to-day care in your town. It could also be helpful to talk to the hospital and practice administrators about expanding pediatric sleep options in the community. In a situation where there's a local hospital but most people go to the bigger city for treatment, smaller hospitals are often looking for a way to "keep patients local." Partnering with them for your sleep dentistry program could help both your practice and their hospital.

If You're in a Bigger City

If you're finding that the physicians you approach already have preferred providers for pediatric sleep dentistry, look for people who are new to the area and only recently opened their practices, or people who are aggressively advertising that they're seeking new patients and trying to expand. Frankly, you don't need the oldest or most experienced physician to diagnose your pediatric sleep patients. You've already screened and examined them. You just need a provider who can see the patient, look over the documentation you've provided, and order the sleep study.

Younger, hungrier physicians are more eager to build the kind of relationships you want. Reach out to them. Give them a call or go visit. Talk about how you can help build each other's practices while improving your community's health.

Remembering the 7-Touch Rule of Marketing, and Other Hints

Remember when you were concerned about marketing your program? Here, building relationships with physicians, is where the marketing actually happens. You don't need billboards and newspaper ads to build your relationships with physicians, but you should consider a few principles of marketing:

- **It can take up to 7 marketing "touches" to get a response** - So, meet people at educational events, send postcards and letters, call, email, visit, and...maybe you need one last contact to convince them to respond to you. Remember, your sleep program is a high priority to you, but it is not a high priority to the physicians. You need to build their sense of interest and urgency until it becomes important enough to act on.
- **Be an authority** - To partner with a physician, you need to convince them that you're serious about your program and sleep dentistry. Learn the science and medicine backing up your program. Be ready to talk about it. Get out in the community as a sleep evangelist so that you have a reputation as a serious practitioner of sleep medicine who cares about patient lives. Make it clear that you can pull your weight in this partnership, you're not just along for the ride.
- **Be likeable** - People want to partner with people they like. So be friendly and warm. Be helpful. Be considerate and willing to say "thank you for your help." You can even ask for advice. You want your physician network to be happy when they hear from you. If you're unsure how to do this without going too far and becoming an annoyance, ask a good friend for advice.

- **Leverage reciprocity** - People are hard-wired to reciprocate favors. So, send a little swag (like note pads). Send over a few test referrals. Invite your prospective physicians to educational luncheons where you provide the food. Drop off treats for their office teams along with your contact info.

I know we all got into this field to become excellent clinicians and to improve our communities. Building these relationships can feel strange and uncomfortable – we're dentists, not realtors or drug reps. Even if you're nervous, keep working on these person-to-person connections. They're what you have to do now so that you can get the kids in your practice the care they need.

Implementation on Target!

After this chapter you should:

- Have at least 1-2 pediatric ENTs who you want to reach
- Find the names of area SLPs and OTS, both in and out of the school system, who might be interested in learning more
- Compile a list of other specialists to introduce yourself to
- Be able to outline an educational program for Physicians and other professionals, about pediatric sleep medicine, the role a sleep dentist plays, and how to help these kids
- Draft a letter of introduction to explain yourself and your program
- Send that letter to the providers on your list

Source for Chapter 14:

https://www.aadsm.org/docs/State_Dental_Board_HSAT_Chart_2021.pdf

15: Should You Add Myofunctional Therapy To Your Practice?

In this chapter you will learn:

- What myofunctional therapy is
- How it can help your sleep patients, both pediatric and adult
- How someone can train in myofunctional therapy
- Ways to add a myofunctional therapist to your team
- How to incorporate myofunctional therapy into sleep dentistry appointments
- Alternatives to adding myofunctional therapy in the office

So far, we've been focused on underlying physical causes of OSA in children, like enlarged tonsils and adenoids, high and narrow palates, blocked sinuses, and unrevised tongue ties. However, even after you correct the underlying physical problems, there will still be issues of ***habit and muscle training.***

While a child's airway is blocked, he develops coping strategies to make breathing possible. These are good under the circumstances – they keep air flowing! But they're not good long-term habits, and once we've cleared the obstruction we need to retrain the muscles of the face and throat to support healthy breathing. In fact, training the muscles before treatment can result in better treatment outcomes. This is where myofunctional therapy can multiply the good effects of other interventions for even better sleep outcomes.

Learning more about myofunctional was amazing. There had always been "chokey" kids in my practice, who choked or gagged on many foods and whose mothers were desperately asking me, their dentist, for help in teaching them to chew and swallow better. And yes, a lot of these kids were also my sleep patients! Knowing about this extra piece that could make treatment more effective and have a wider impact on their daily lives was amazing! This was something my patients and their parents needed, and no one else was offering it to them.

What is Myofunctional Therapy (MFT)?

The muscles in the face, mouth, and throat all work together for breathing, swallowing, speaking, and chewing. When someone is a full or partial mouth breather, these muscles stop working well together. This impacts their sleep breathing but also impacts their speech and their chewing and swallowing. Children with unreleased tongue ties don't learn to use all these muscles efficiently. Neither do children who are habitual mouth breathers.

The therapy works on strengthening these muscles and retraining them to work together. The therapist works with the patient in an office setting, and then gives them personalized exercises to perform at home. A good therapist has several protocols and then adjusts them for individual patients and their practices.

How Does MFT Help Pediatric (and Even Adult!) Sleep Patients?

Very young children often learn age-appropriate orofacial motor movements within days or a few weeks of a tongue-tie release. However, older children have had longer to develop bad habits and need more time and effort to retrain their muscles. While they ***can*** do this on their own, they can achieve good function more quickly by completing a therapy program.

Myofunctional therapy can also help before tongue and lip ties are released. For some children with "looser ties," the therapy alone is enough to reduce their sleep breathing issues, support nasal breathing, and encourage a close-mouthed posture.

For other children, especially older children, a series of myofunctional therapy sessions before a scheduled tongue or lip-tie release makes the surgery less painful and traumatic, speeds healing and gives them the skills and muscle tone they need so that they can quickly catch up developmentally.

Since every aspect of our – speaking, eating, learning, socializing – depends on the ability to breathe well, the sooner we can correct these issues, the sooner children can make up for lost time and catch up with their age-mates.

MFT also results in better outcomes when used in conjunction with appliances. Our kids aren't wearing these appliances all day, just when they sleep and for an hour or so more. At school, at sports, even watching TV, it's easy to fall into the habit of mouth breathing again. OMFT supports nasal breathing all day, while our appliances support it at night. The daytime component is especially important when they're eating or drinking.

When you start a therapy program in your office, you get better outcomes, these kids get back in the swing of school and life more quickly, they're able to eat a better and more balanced diet, and they are also getting better rest. They can be a part of how our sleep programs support the whole health of the child.

What Training Do We Need to Offer Myofunctional Therapist?

There are two kinds of myofunctional therapists. A trained therapist is someone who has completed a class in myofunctional therapy and who has begun diagnosing and treating patients. Various providers offer these courses. In a myofunctional therapy class one generally learns:

- How the muscles of the mouth, face, and throat work together to support healthy breathing, chewing, swallowing, and speaking.
- How to identify dysfunctions of these muscles and more muscle tone.
- Which exercises can be used to improve function, how to teach them, and how to track a patient's progress.
- How to talk to patients and their families about myofunctional therapy.

Some courses may also discuss payment, insurance, and how to set up a therapy schedule for a patient.

A *certified* therapist has also completed additional requirements and has received certification from an official organization. Several organizations certify oral-myofunctional therapists, and the certifications carry equal weight in the field.

To be a certified therapist, you must first be in one of the allowable occupations. In a typical dental office, either dentists or registered dental hygienists can train for therapy. Speech and language pathologists, occupational therapists, physical therapists, and chiropractors can also be certified.

To get full certification, the therapist must also

- Complete a certain number of cases overseen by a certified mentor
- Complete case studies for a certain number of patients treated
- Pass a certification exam

Certification does not affect billing for myofunctional therapy services, but some providers find it helps attract patients. Since you'll be offering myofunctional therapy to your existing pediatric sleep patients, certification is not usually necessary.

How Can I Offer Myofunctional Therapy to My Patients?

The easiest way to offer myofunctional therapy to your patients is to have someone on the team who can act as a therapist. To do this you can:

- Hire a hygienist who is already trained
- Take the training yourself
- Help one of your current RDHs get trained

A second option is to work with an outside therapist who is a myofunctional therapist and who can come in and offer therapy on certain days of the month or remotely. Then you can schedule sleep follow-up appointments for those days and have patients complete therapy in-office.

Finally, you can refer patients to an outside therapist with whom you've established a relationship, such as an OT or SLP. The one drawback here is that your patients may not be willing to attend extra appointments at a strange office.

What Does Myofunctional Therapy in a Dental Office Look Like?

In my office, I usually see patients for about 8-12 sessions, before and after they have tongue and lip ties revised. This is usually enough to help them build muscle tone and learn how to breathe and swallow well. However, each case and the number of sessions needed is based upon the patients' needs as determined clinically and after a detailed evaluation. Older children and adults may be more diligent about completing the exercises and need fewer sessions. If a child has lower muscle tone or motor planning issues, he may need more sessions.

At an appointment, I check my patient's progress, then work with them on a new set of exercises to help them keep advancing. I send my patients home with homework and have them mark down how many exercises they're completing. I prefer parents to watch as I show exercises to their children so they can support proper form at home.

Myofunctional therapy can sometimes help children avoid T&A surgery or a CPAP. Once we enable and support nasal breathing, inflamed tonsils and adenoids sometimes heal – they're often a *symptom* of bad breathing habits, not the cause of them. By treating the root causes and helping get the tongue in the proper position, the mouth closed, and the airway clear, we can change lives with myofunctional therapy.

After learning about orofacial myofunctional therapy, I trained as a therapist and got certified. Once I was certified, I encouraged my RDH to get trained too. This therapy modality is so useful, not just for our sleep patients, but also for our TMJ patients, and it's really helped our practice grow.

Implementation on Target!

After this chapter you should:

- Consider whether orofacial myotherapy is right for your practice
- Investigate courses yourself or choose an RDH who is willing to take the courses
- Develop a plan for using myofunctional therapy as part of your tongue and lip tie revision program

16: Tongue-Tie, Palate Expansion, and Habit-Trainers

In this chapter you will learn:

- About steps to take before deciding on a course of treatment
- How to choose different appliances depending on patient needs
- Start identifying the appliances that will work best in your practice

As you begin to screen and treat sleep patients, you'll notice that a large number of these kids have issues with tongue ties, lip ties, and high narrow palates. That's because craniofacial development has a huge impact on the airway. When a child's airway is obstructed, there are a few steps we should follow so that they get the maximum benefit from our care.

A T&A is often just a Band-Aid. Yes, the tonsils and adenoids are swollen and making it harder for the child to breathe, but they are swollen because the child is not practicing nasal breathing. When we correct the craniofacial issues and posture issues, the child can breathe normally and then the tonsils and adenoids return to normal without unnecessary surgery.

Initially, I'd send my patients to an ENT who'd do a T&A right out of the gate, since it's generally considered first-line treatment for sleep breathing issues. And they'd be fine for a year or two, and then they'd have the same issues all over again. T&A was just not helping.

Once I learned about craniofacial development and the airway, I realized where I'd been going wrong. We have to fix the palate, the tongue, and the nasal cavity if we want lasting change.

So, what should your goals be for these patients?

1. Clear the nose and sinuses so that nasal breathing is possible. Often these kids have untreated allergies or sinus infections that have made it hard for them to breathe through their noses.
2. Retrain the child in close-lipped nasal breathing. Strengthen and train the tongue and the cheek muscles.
3. If needed, free the tongue. For some children, the myofunctional therapy will be enough to correct their issues, but for most, they will also need a tongue or lip-tie release. As we discussed in the last chapter, this procedure is more effective if it is both preceded and followed by myofunctional therapy.
4. Finally, after the tongue has healed, see if expanding the palate is necessary and beneficial. Decide on an appliance and protocol based on the degree of expansion needed.

Why do I focus so much on the maxilla and its role in facial development? Because the roof of the mouth is the floor of the nasal cavity. When that floor is broad and flat, there's more room for free movement of air. Colds or allergies don't result in total blockages, it's possible to clear the nose and drain the sinuses.

If, on the other hand, that floor is like the top of a high, narrow arch, you don't get a free flow of air. It's harder to clear the nose and sinuses. The child becomes a mouth-breather, with all the problems that result.

To repeat, because the roof of the mouth is the floor of the nasal cavity. The maxilla matters.

In very young children, the tongue can act as a natural palate expander as well as a retainer. Once any ties are released and the child learns to habitually rest the tongue on the roof of the mouth, the maxilla might develop normally on its own. But in older children and adults, appliances and sometimes even surgery can be necessary to support proper nasal breathing.

In this section, I'll be discussing some of my favorite appliances for supporting proper facial growth so that the airway stays open. I'm not affiliated with any of these companies, but these are the appliances that have worked best in my practice.

Habit Correctors

Habit correctors are wonderful for small children who have had a tongue tie released or who developed a habit of mouth-breathing after nasal blockage from colds or allergies.

A good habit corrector teaches the child to breathe with tightly closed lips, trains them to rest their tongue on the roof of the mouth, and helps the cheek and facial muscles support speaking and chewing. These are great appliances. In fact, if you have a kid with lower muscle tone as a toddler, habit correction can head off finicky eating, gagging, and speech articulation issues down the road.

In my practice, I sometimes use the Healthy Start System. Their habit corrector can take anywhere from one to six months to work, and most toddlers and young preschoolers tolerate it well.

Another system we've had good luck with is the Myobrace system, as well as the Myomunchies for very young children. These both correct bad habits and clean the teeth, and many children prefer them to pacifiers, so they're a good, healthy substitution that sets them up for a lifetime of health.

Orthotropics, Not Orthodontics

For older kids, many of the appliances we use are orthotropics, not orthodontics. This means that the focus isn't just on straight teeth, but on proper facial development. This leads to straighter teeth and a better smile, but it also leads to a flatter, wider maxilla, a more open nasal cavity, and easier breathing.

Does a child's palate need expanding? Look at how far off the width of the upper arch is from the ideal width.

The benefits of palate expansion include a decrease in nasal resistance, better support for nasal breathing, improved speech and eating, more room for the adult teeth as they abrupt, and ultimately a better smile. We're expanding the airway and training the muscles so that they'll be able to breathe and sleep well into adulthood, and we may be preventing future OSA or UARS.

TOTS Before Expansion

For my patients, I usually deal with any tethered oral tissues (TOTS) in conjunction with MFT before expansion. Freeing up that tongue and lip make breathing and eating instantly better, and it helps them benefit more from the palate expansion. The tongue and the palate work together in sleep breathing, speech, and eating, so both the tongue and the palate must be healthy.

Releasing ties is fairly fast and the children show immediate improvement. Expanding the palate takes longer. It doesn't make sense to leave tethered oral tissue until the palate work is complete. Do it first.

I cannot say enough about how changing my philosophy on tethered tongues changed the lives of my patients. I'm not just correcting sleep issues. I'm also helping them speak, eat, and feel more confident. These kids have been ill-served by wait-and-see on tongue ties. It's time to help them.

Why Tethered Tongues Cause Big Problems

Most pediatricians only revise the most severe tethered tongues – those that are keeping a child from eating enough to grow. But even less severe tethers can cause big issues like:

- A high narrow palate because the tongue should act as a natural palate expander and can't.
- Vastly shortened nursing time, because nursing a baby with a tethered tongue is hard and painful for the mother.
- Sleep-disordered breathing, because a low tongue cannot rest up in the palate. Instead, it flops backward and impinges on the oropharyngeal area.
- Problems moving food around the mouth while eating. This results in chokey kids, kids with reflux, kids with very restricted food choices, and an increased risk of tooth decay.
- Speech and language issues. The child cannot articulate well because he cannot move his tongue. His parents and peers can't understand him. When it's time to learn to read, he has trouble with phonics because to him many letter sounds all seem to be the same.

As newborn frenectomies have become less common, we're seeing more and more older kids coming to our practice with these issues. One of the best things we can do for them is to release those ties and get them the range of movement they need to be healthy.

Practices can use either a laser frenectomy or surgery with a scalpel or surgical scissors to release the ties. Both procedures have benefits and drawbacks.

Laser Frenectomy

The benefits of Laser Frenectomy are that it is fast, easy, and can be done with a topical-only anesthetic. The drawbacks are that there is often more scarring if done improperly, which can impede movement or cause discomfort later. It's also more likely to result in an incomplete release of the tie.

Surgery

The downsides of surgery are that it takes longer than a laser, requires local anesthesia, uses sutures, and also takes more practice.

It also minimizes scarring and allows you to remove the scar tissue from previous, incomplete releases.

Measuring the Palate

After the tongue tie has been released and the child has healed from surgery, it's time to evaluate the palate. Since they haven't been able to rest their tongue in the roof of their mouth, they are going to need expansion. The question is simply how much expansion.

I like to use both the Schwarz Index and the Ponts Number when planning treatment. The two numbers give me slightly different information and give me a clearer picture of what appliances will be best for this child. I highly recommend that you purchase a Boley gauge for these measurements and learn to use it. It's much more accurate than a straight measure, and better measurements mean better results.

Quick Review of the Schwarz Index (SI)

This is a quick reminder of how to find the Schwarz Index and expansion needs for your patient. If this is new to you, take a class on this topic.

- Find the mesiodistal width of each of the four upper incisors, and add those measurements together. This number is the SI
- Measure the actual width of the arch at the first premolar, and record it.
- Compute the ideal width, which is the SI+8. Record that.
- The difference between actual and ideal is the need for expansion at the first premolar.
- Now measure the actual width at the molars. Record this number.
- Compute the ideal width, SI + 16. Record that number.
- The difference between actual and ideal is the need for expansion at the molars.

The younger we catch these kids, the sooner we can get that palate where it needs to be as they grow. However, if you don't release the tongue first, you lose that natural palate expansion action, and they're more likely to need a second round of expansion later. So again, first the tongue, then expand.

Other Measurements

I like the ***Ponts index*** because it adds a few more dimensions that give insight into a child's facial development needs. If the child's anterior triangle measurement is off, you may want to use a 3-way appliance instead of a 2-way.

The ***Mew Indicator Line*** Measures the distance from the tip of the nose to the incisors and can also help you develop a plan for supporting good facial development as the child grows.

Implementation On Target!

After this chapter, you should:

- Develop a plan and a checklist for helping patients clear out those nasal cavities
- Understand and be able to explain to parents why OMT can help establish nasal breathing and heal the tonsils and adenoids
- Develop your frenectomy protocol
- Get a Boley gauge, if you didn't already have one
- Learn to confidently measure and compute Schwarz numbers, Ponts Numbers, and Mews Numbers
- Choose the appliances and treatment protocols that work best for your practice

17: Setting Up Your Pedo Funnel in the Office

In this chapter, you will learn how to:

- **Identify key parts of an in-office pediatric sleep funnel**
- **Begin to plan your funnel**
- **Decide which materials you'll use to support your funnel**
- **Develop team roles in the funnel**

Initially, I worried about how I'd talk to parents about our new sleep program. I'd seen how revolutionary it was for my own family, and I wanted to help as many of my patients as possible, but I was worried about seeming pushy. Setting up a good in-office funnel meant that people were ready for these conversations long before I opened my mouth.

Your in-office funnel is the way that current pediatric dental patients and their parents will learn about your sleep program and become interested. So that, by the time you see them for their examination, they are ready and willing to hear what you'll have to tell them about pediatric sleep and their child's symptoms.

In marketing, a funnel helps guide people to saying yes to a product. It starts out with a wide array of vary shallow information, and then, as people go deeper, the focus narrows. At each step, the funnel nudges the shopper to the next step. Not every shopper goes from "site visit" to "purchase" on every visit, but because marketing is about multiple touches, when they return to a site they'll often start at the point where they left the funnel, not back at the beginning.

The same goes for the pediatric sleep funnel in your office. Parents may not be willing to take action on their child's sleep issues after a single visit. It might seem too new, or the family may have other things going on that make tackling another round of appointments difficult. However, given enough time, most parents will be ready to get their children help – you just have to plant those seeds, and you can plant those seeds at every step of their journey through your office.

Pediatric Sleep Funnel Basics

Some of the points in your pediatric sleep funnel that need special attention are:

- Your social media/direct email
- The appointment reminder call/mailing/text
- At check-in
- Your waiting area and restroom
- On the way to the patient bay
- In the patient bay
- At checkout
- After the appointment

Your Social Media and Email Lists

Social media and email lists are an excellent way to pique parental interest in pediatric sleep dentistry. Include sleep medicine posts or updates in your normal rounds of online communications. Celebrate patients who are helped, mention symptoms of sleep apnea or tongue and lip ties, and let parents know that you can evaluate their kids for these conditions.

Up to 10% of children may have unrevised tongue and lip ties, so chances are that some of the parents reading your updates will recognize their child. Often, parents need to think about a diagnosis or procedure for a while before they'll take action. Social media nudges start the idea percolating so that by the time the family sees you they're ready to take action on sleep apnea.

I was surprised by how responsive parents were to my social media posts and emails about pediatric sleep medicine. This was something new, not just reminding them about healthy eating or oral hygiene, and they were excited! My new service was solving a problem that many parents had, and that no one was offering help for.

The Appointment Reminders

Whether you connect with your patients by phone, text, email, or good old-fashioned snail mail, the appointment reminder is a great time to stir up a bit of interest in your sleep program. Just add a line that at the beginning of the appointment, parents will create a sleep screening form for their children. You can even pull out a few sample questions if you have space and time.

This prepares parents for a new form at check-in and gets them to start looking for signs of poor sleeping in their kids. Since recall on the spot is sometimes poor, if parents spend longer looking for signs, you'll get more accurate results from your screening tools.

At Check-In

At Check-In, have your front office team remind parents that you're screening children for sleep issues, palate problems, and tongue and lip ties. During the check-in process, have the parents fill out a sleep screening along with the other health forms.

Your desk team should specifically thank the parents for filling out the sleep screen. If they have any questions about the new program, the team should be able to answer them and give examples of how the new program helps kids with behavior, academic, and social problems.

Hang a "Why are we screening for pediatric sleep issues?" flier where patients can see it as they check-in. Most won't stop to read it, but even having it there will make the sleep program seem more familiar to parents.

In the Waiting Area

Seed the waiting area with information on the pediatric sleep program. For instance, books and magazines focused on kids and sleep, pamphlets about tongue-ties and how they affect kids, videos playing about sleep and sleep interventions.

For instance, you may want a short segment that airs demonstrating the basics of myofunctional therapy, or another showing what tongue and lip ties look like. The more familiar parents are with your program before their child is in the chair, the more comfortable they'll be discussing sleep.

As with the adult program, it's helpful to have posters with QR codes for parents who may want to dig deeper. Some of the parents will be utterly indifferent to the sleep program – they're here to hear "Look, Ma, No Cavities!" and get out. Others will see how sleep may be the thread connecting their child's issues, and they'll be excited and eager to learn more.

Again, as with adult information, the restroom is an ideal place to post quick information about sleep, because it's one place where people will actually take time to read what's on the walls.

On the Walk Back to the Operatory

The walk back to the patient operatory is another place to advertise your pediatric sleep program. Bulletin boards, posters, and proclamations of the number of kids you've gotten to sleep better all help parents understand that your program is here to help kids just like theirs. By this point in the appointment, many of the parents will be curious about the sleep program.

In the Patient Op

When parents are in the patient op, they spend a lot of time sitting and looking at things. Take advantage of this! More posters, models of the tongue, palate, and throat, and pamphlets can keep parents thinking about sleep dentistry.

During the hygiene portion of the appointment, the hygienist should be prepared to answer questions, or at least to pass those questions on to you before your examination begins. If any of your hygienists have seen their own children helped by sleep dentistry, encourage them to talk to patients about their family's experiences. If there is a child who you suspect, even before the appointment, may have sleep issues, try to assign them to the hygienists who are most excited about the new program.

At Checkout

At the checkout desk, send parents home with information about pediatric sleep dentistry, tips for good sleep hygiene, and a coloring sheet or activity book for the kids. Include an extra card or brochure and encourage parents to refer a friend whose child may need an evaluation. If they had a good appointment and are excited about what they learned, encourage them to make a social post. You can even have a "pedo sleep photo spot" set up so that parents and kids can have fun taking a goofy picture to promote pediatric sleep screening.

After the Appointment

After a child's checkup, follow up with a postcard, email, or call to see if the parent has any further questions about sleep dentistry. If you made referrals to other offices, follow up about those as well. Even if this first appointment didn't get a parent to take action, you've planted the seeds. In six months, when the family returns, you can always bring it up again in your chat with the parent.

Follow-up has been helpful for us. So many parents walk out with "I'll have to think about this." Gentle nudges in the months after the appointment mean that they actually take the time to think and research after they leave the office. Otherwise, they forget because life is busy and they're used to the status quo.

Pediatric Funnel FAQ

Is it harder to set up a funnel than you expected? Here are some common questions about pediatric sleep funnels.

Where Are All the Waiting Room Materials Going?

If people keep walking off with your waiting room materials about children and sleep, you must be doing something right. You picked reading material that was interesting and engaging enough that parents want to spend more time with it. One way to prevent that is to label copies "Waiting Area Only" but have a sign offering copies to take home. When you give a parent a "take home" copy of a book or magazine, record who it was (you can contact them later about their child) and encourage them to pass it on when they're done reading. Make sure a sticker with your office info is prominently displayed on any "loaner" materials so that if they get passed hand to hand, parents can find you and get help for their kids.

Parents Seem Shocked When I Bring up Tongue and Palate Issues During my Examination. Why?

This suggests that they aren't aware and/or your materials aren't doing a good enough job connecting sleep and behavior issues to physical issues in the mouth. One way to improve this is to add a supplement to your sleep screening materials that ask about things like feeding behaviors as an infant (If they nursed, was it painful? Did they seem glued to the breast? Did they chomp down a lot? Were they slow to grow? If they bottle-fed, were they slow eaters? Were they gassy? Did they have reflux?) and as toddlers and young kids (Are they fussy eaters? Do they choke or gag a lot? Do they avoid certain textures? Are they slow eaters? Do they need SLP services, especially for L, R, C, and S sounds?) When you add these sorts of questions to your screenings, it's easier to explain why tongues and palates matter so much for sleep and behavior.

I Keep Seeing Kids Who Need Help, But Their Parents are Reluctant to Say Yes to Treatment. What Can I do to Help?

When parents are reluctant to say yes to treatment for their kids, there are usually a few underlying causes:

- They're worried that it will be unaffordable.
- They're worried it will be painful or dangerous to their child.
- They're worried that they won't have the time to come to appointments, either because of work schedules, school/activity schedules, or the needs of other family members.
- They need time to research and develop an opinion.

It might be worthwhile for you to have a handout prepared for parents addressing these concerns and add it to the waiting room reading material or pre-appointment paperwork. Be clear about the risks of untreated sleep apnea versus the risks of treatment. Provide them with links and references. Explain how many appointments/how much time in the chair it takes to produce a lasting benefit.

Parents want to help their kids be healthy, happy, and successful. But they're also juggling a host of worries and concerns, so be compassionate and supportive. They'll get to "yes," it just takes some time to make mental space for treatment.

My Team is Still Skeptical of Sleep Dentistry, and I Think They're Passing that on to the Patients

I love my team. They're great people. But it took them a little while to come around to pediatric sleep dentistry because it was a new kind of dentistry for them. Clear aligners made sense. That's dentist stuff. They were fine with mouth guards for athletes. We care about teeth! But bringing in the airway confused them.

I found I had to do a lot more education with them to persuade them that we weren't getting out of our lane and that we were qualified to handle airway issues. Once I persuaded them that this was something that fell under our specialty, the skepticism faded fast. They just needed to be sure that we were good enough and skilled enough to do right by these kids.

If your team is still skeptical, you started the program too soon and didn't engage them enough in the process. Identify one or two key members to undergo sleep training, and see if they have anyone in their own lives who could benefit from pediatric sleep dentistry. Your team needs to see that someone they know and trust has personal experience with the benefits that come from treating these kids. Once they see that first "cure," they'll be excited because they'll have concrete evidence that this is a program that changes lives.

If you have certain team members who persist in undermining your pediatric program and disrupting your in-office funnels, you have a few options:

- Train them more
- Move them out of patient-facing positions, or at least out of pediatric patient-facing positions
- Recognize that they're a poor fit for your office and culture at this time

That said, I have found that *almost every single person* can get excited about pediatric sleep dentistry once they see how the airway is connected to all other parts of life, and how greatly airway issues can impact child development. So, in most cases, these sorts of negative comments really are the result of "not enough education at a level the team member can understand." Or, sometimes, guilt, if the team member sees their own child's struggles in these children, and regrets not having helped them. In either case, honest conversations and listening can go a long way to changing team members' minds.

Setting up good sleep funnels is an important part of your pediatric program. You're doing life-changing work in your office, and parents need to know that help is available for their kids.

Implementation on Target!

At the end of this chapter you should:

- Update your pre-appointment and check-in paperwork to include sleep information
- Add pediatric sleep dentistry to the rotation for your blog, social media, and email blasts
- Make a diagram of your office and how a patient moves through it. Identify where you can use the space to assist your sleep funnel
- Decide where you're getting your educational materials for the office. Is a current team member making them? Are you downloading from your sleep course and rebranding? Are you hiring someone to produce them? Are you purchasing books and posters?
- Talk to team members about their roles in the sleep funnel, and how to integrate pediatric sleep dentistry into their normal interactions with patients

18: Community Outreach for Pediatric Sleep

In this chapter you'll learn:

- How to do community outreach
- Which platforms are best for educating your community about pediatric airway dentistry
- How to tailor your message for different audiences in the community

I was pretty busy just with the kids in my practice, and word of mouth was bringing us new patients, but I wanted to do more. As I saw the real change we were making in these kids' lives, my heart ached for the kids whose parents didn't know about the effects of poor sleep, the kids who were being labeled bad, or hyperactive, or slow at school, when really, they just needed to get that airway open and breathe.

Pediatric sleep dentistry is a much-needed service in our communities, and many parts of the country still don't have access to pediatric sleep dentists. This has huge effects on kids. They're not succeeding, they're on meds to cope with psychiatric issues arising from an obstructed airway, and they're living with other complications from the tongue and palate issues underlying it all.

Your program will grow without advertising (Parental word of mouth is powerful) but it's still worthwhile to go out into the community and teach parents, teachers, therapists, and physicians about pediatric sleep breathing. Why? When you reach out and educate, you're not just helping with the physical side of things. You're helping these kids get the recognition and compassion they need from the adults around them. You're changing lives and ensuring that every parent has access to the information they need to help their children.

If you're used to hanging back and avoiding the spotlight, you don't need to do this all at once, or all that often. I'd just like to outline some of the ways that you can help spread the word about pediatric airway dentistry and what it can do for these kids. No one educates in all of these places and ways. Pick the ones that fit best with your community and your personality.

Also, you do still have your clinical work. So, if community education won't fit into your schedule, it's fine to delegate it to a team member who loves teaching and understands pediatric airway dentistry. But I would urge you to take a lead role in at least some of this community education – it's rewarding and a great way to reach new audiences while changing lives.

Where to Educate

Every community has organizations that need guest educators. Here are a few to consider as you give back to the community by educating about pediatric airways and sleep.

Health Fairs

Find out when your local health organizations have their annual health fairs, and consider getting a table. This is a way for you, or your team, to have in-person, one-on-one conversations about how the palate and tongue affect children's health. Bring models and other educational equipment for people to look at and touch. These events let you give back to the community by providing education and information to parents, grandparents, and educators.

Back to School Nights

Does your community have back-to-school nights with tables from local groups? Show up! It's a way to support the school while teaching parents and teachers about airways and sleep breathing. Remember, most people have not heard about pediatric sleep apnea, palate issues, or how breathing, eating, and speaking are all intertwined! You have interesting and helpful information to share, and getting out there into your local school communities can make a big difference.

Health Classes

Have you considered giving guest lectures at the local high school or community college? Students training for careers in health sciences are an excellent group for your outreach. These students are eager to learn about health issues, and you can provide them a perspective they might not otherwise get. When you reach out to these classes, you teach students who will go on and share their knowledge with their families and future patients. A little effort can amplify your message about airways and sleep.

Going into classes is very rewarding for me. I get to speak to young people just starting out in the health field, and teach them something new. Sometimes, they recognize themselves, siblings, or children in the profile of a child with airway issues. Other times, they leave that class as sleep and airway evangelists, inspired to save lives and make a difference. Really, everyone should guest lecture at least once. It's such a good experience, and these young people are eager to learn.

Scouting Organizations, 4H, and the YMCA

These groups are also always looking for people to come in and talk about health and wellness topics. Teaching teens about healthy sleep and breathing can have a huge impact on them, their parents, and their siblings. Again, this is a great way to give back, by teaching future leaders why sleep is a priority.

Groups like the Kiwanis, Chamber of Commerce, or Hospital Auxiliary

Many local community groups have lunch or breakfast meetings where they host speakers. Volunteering to present about pediatric sleep issues is a great way to educate community leaders who will take this information home to their children and grandchildren.

Teacher In-Service Days

Schools are often at a loss to provide educational programming to their teachers on in-service days, and sometimes have local pediatricians and dentists in to give programs related to child health and development. These in-service days are a wonderful opportunity, because teachers see kids every day with airway issues, and they may not be aware of them. Instead, they're seeing signs of ADHD, laziness, Oppositional Defiant Disorder, low energy, speech issues, sensory issues, and poor posture. Teaching the teachers about the possibility of underlying physical causes means that these kids will get more understanding and compassion at school and be more likely to get help for underlying issues at home. Again, you don't need to do outreach to grow your sleep dentistry program, but outreach means that you save more kids.

Nurse, Physician and Therapists Study Groups

Most areas have study groups for medical professionals. Contact hospitals and local professional organizations, and offer to give presentations. You have valuable information that can help other professionals serve children. The more that you're out and seen in the community, teaching about these things, the more professionals will be aware of the issues and understand that help is available.

Local Newspapers and Lifestyle Magazines

Both of these are usually desperate for content, so if you enjoy writing, this is a great way to educate your community. Even though most busy parents rarely read the paper or these magazines, grandparents do. And grandparents can be great allies when it comes to helping kids get the medical help they need to learn, socialize, and be happy.

Local Television and Radio, Especially Morning Shows

If you're in a mid-to-large-sized city, morning shows are a great way to educate people in the community. Parents and grandparents watch these as they get the kids through their morning routine and out the door, and the shows themselves are often desperate for guests to fill airtime. If you like the camera, speak well, and want to do your part to educate your community about pediatric airway issues, this is the platform for you. You can send a letter or press release about what you do and offering to appear, and follow up with a phone call. If it's a good experience for you and the studio team, you may even get regular call-backs. And, even if you decide TV isn't for you, that first appearance will help kids.

Radio is also an option, especially the local "80s/90s and Today" station. Local stations will sometimes have guests and discuss issues that impact their listeners, and you could catch some parents or teachers on the drive to school and work.

How to Educate: Knowing Your Audience

The first step to being an excellent pediatric airway dentistry educator is to know your audience. Who are you talking to? Are you speaking to other medical professionals, to teachers and other people who work with children, or to parents and grandparents? If you're using mass media, who watches or reads? Each group will benefit from a different approach, ask different types of questions, and have a different goal as they learn about pediatric airway dentistry.

The biggest challenge when I started doing community outreach was navigating the different audiences. I couldn't talk to a physician's roundtable the same way I talked to a morning show host. I got better with practice, and I found that doing this outreach also made me a better educator in the office too!

For Medical Professionals

Teaching other medical professionals about airway dentistry can be incredibly rewarding, but also very challenging. With this group, you can be very technical. You'll need to bring all your research and statistics and examples from studies. But you also need to expect to be challenged more with this group. You're on their turf, and they're going to want to put you to the test before they seriously consider what you have to say. Here are a few hints to help those first few talks go smoothly.

- **Start with your credentials** - Let your audience know where you were educated, if you did residencies, and what specialties you have. It's important for them to know, out of the gate, that you're practicing real medicine, this isn't just "woo-woo."
- **Get technical, bring diagrams** - Get technical. Talk about the anatomical issues underlying sleep breathing, the conditions this can cause, and how to solve them. Go into details about the surgery you perform and why it's helpful. This audience will understand what you tell them, and they won't respect you if you talk down to them.
- **Be ready with research and studies** - Even if it sounds good, you need evidence. In fact, it might be helpful to have either a webpage they can visit or a handout listing where to find the relevant studies supporting your sleep dentistry program.
- **If you have case studies, bring them** - Who have you actually helped? What were the results? Were there any side effects?
- **Expect lots of specific questions** - The questions might be the most stressful part of educating other medical professionals. So lean into them! This is a chance for you to learn and improve your skills too.
- **Have fun!** When you educate medical professionals it's a chance to meet with people who are as passionate about pediatric care as you are. You might not all agree on the importance of the airway, but this is your chance to plant

seeds, and also a chance to get out of the office and learn things about your own field through the lens of other fields.

For Teachers, Caregivers, and Other Professionals Who Work With Children

You can't use the same presentation you've developed for medical professionals with teachers and other non-medical professionals who work with children. For one, they won't easily grasp your anatomical and technical vocabulary. In the second place, their concerns are different. They aren't wondering, "How is this procedure done and what are the risks," as much as, "How can I help my students adjust to the classroom and grasp grade-level material?" That means that you're going to have to shift your language and your focus to talk to this group.

You would not believe the stories teachers tell once you get them talking. Some of these kids have SO MANY PROBLEMS, but since no one has looked at their airways, they just get labeled as bad kids. It's such a relief to educators when they realize there's help available. They knew the doctors must be missing something, and now they know what the missing piece is and can start connecting these tough students with real help.

- **Only use technical language in their areas of specialty** - If you're talking about ADHD, ODD, or other learning and behavioral disorders related to sleep apnea, this audience will understand the acronyms. But they're not as steeped in medical terminology as you are, so when it comes to the anatomy and physiology of sleep dentistry, talk to them like parents, not like physicians.
- **Focus on the aspects of airway dentistry that matter most for them and the children they work with** - For teachers and other adults who work with children, prime concerns are going to be behavior, learning, and social skills. How does this disorder impact a child's ability to succeed in the classroom? Why do other interventions fail if the underlying issue has

not been treated? How do speech/language issues and feeding difficulties affect the school day?

- **Give them the tools to talk to parents** - When these professionals suspect that a child may have an underlying tongue, palate, or breathing issue, they need tools to talk to parents about who they can see and where they can get an evaluation. One reason the T&A is the first line for all children is that, in many communities, no practitioner is treating the underlying tongue and palate issues. Make sure they know where to go to get help, and that you're willing to look at the students who need help.
- **Take time to listen** - In this group, questions are often of the form of, "I have this student and..." They both want advice on how to help these kids *and* a friendly and compassionate listener. Kids with sleep issues create a real struggle for educators, and teachers often aren't heard when they insist there must be something else going on with a kid. You have a solution, but there's a lot of emotion when someone finds out that there is actually help for these struggling kids.
- **Have handouts ready, and bring models** - When you're teaching teachers, it helps to have models, handouts, and other support materials. They'll respect you more if you take the time to give a really good presentation because teaching is their area of expertise!

For Parents and Grandparents

Unless you're at an event targeted to medical professionals or teaching professionals, most of the time your audience is going to be parents and grandparents. This is true whether you're on television, at a health fair, or somewhere else in the community. Parents and grandparents are an important group to educate because they are the ones who are closest to these kids and most likely to move heaven and earth to get them help. When you're speaking to parents and grandparents, either through media or in person, it's important to remember that you're speaking to a diverse group. They all have different experiences with education, dental and medical care, and how society treats their kids. For this group, compassion is key and has to come before information and authority when you're educating them.

Before you talk to parents or grandparents about airway dentistry, be aware. Some of these parents are going to start bawling as you describe what sleep issues can do to kids and what these kids look like – how they're so painful and exhausting to nurse, hard to understand when speaking, fussy about food, and hard to take out into social issues. These parents have been suffering for so long. They've been feeling like failures because everyone acts like it's a discipline issue, not a sick and hurting kid issue. And now that someone is finally listening, they will cry. Bring a box of tissues to these presentations. They'll get a lot of use.

- **Start with a brief overview of what these kids look like as babies, as toddlers, and as students** - Start at the beginning, and how physical issues can affect breastfeeding and make it impossible for mom. Then talk about speech and feeding issues through infancy and toddlerhood, and finally school and social issues. Mention the posture issues too – these are things many caregivers fight kids over, and can't understand why the kid can't change. When they hear that all of the issues with the child are connected, it's life-changing.
- **If you're in an in-person conversation, get ready to listen** - If you're in person, this is the point where you will be flooded with stories from parents and caregivers. Listen first, then continue educating. Your sympathy and the fact that you're not writing off their kids as "bad kids" or "difficult" will change lives and minds.
- **If you're engaging through TV, radio, or print journalism, give a nod to the fact that many people have had their concerns ignored for years** - Again, this is very traumatic for families. Many have given up seeking help for their kids because they assume that no one in the medical or dental professions will

listen to them. You're listening. They need to know that you understand where they're coming from and are here to help.

- **Explain the physical causes without too much anatomical detail** - You don't need to go into great detail with a general audience. Focus on getting these kids screened. When you describe potential treatments, don't get too gory. Focus on the fact that these are not new or revolutionary procedures, but ones that have fallen out of use. Explain how therapy and exercises can help.
- **Finish off with information on good sleep hygiene** - This is information many parents aren't getting. Also, if you have children of your own, bring in your own experiences of getting kids to sleep and weaning off nighttime devices. Many times, experts give lists of things to do without acknowledging how challenging they are or giving any real tools. You have experience, you have tools. Share them.

Implementation on Target!

After this chapter, you should:

- Identify at least three places where you will educate your community
- Decide whether you or a team member will handle each educational opportunity
- Develop different presentations for medical professionals, teachers, and parents
- Create supporting material as needed
- Reach out and volunteer to do a presentation or teach a class

Conclusion: Are You Ready to Go, or Do You Need More?

Congratulations! You've done some hard work learning about, and planning for, successful implementation of your new sleep programs.

Are you confident and ready to start seeing patients? If not, there are a few areas to take a closer look at:

If You Feel Like There are Still Huge Gaps in Your Knowledge...

Take a look at your education. Have you been to training with an actual sleep dentist, either online or in-person? Or are you trying to implement just based on books and articles? If it's the latter, you may need a course. Sometimes it's less about the information being given and more about the chance to ask questions and get feedback from someone who's been right where you are.

If you have taken a class, try to come up with three concrete questions to ask your instructor! Anyone who has ever tutored knows "I just don't understand!" can cover a huge array of issues. Take the time to formulate a specific question, so that we know where to begin helping you!

If Your Team has Been Trained, But Are Still Confused About What They're Supposed to Be Doing

If your team understands the "why," but not "how" to do it, you need to take a look at systems and checklists, especially related to how patients move through the practice. Make a list of everything that has to happen for both an adult and a pediatric sleep dentistry appointment. Then assign those tasks to team members and create a flowchart and checklist for how your practice will handle these patients.

Make sure everyone in the practice has a copy in their work area so they know both who they are handing tasks off to and who is handing tasks off to them. Eventually, this will become second nature for your team, but at the beginning make sure they have easy to find reference sheets.

If You're Still Reluctant to Talk to Your Patients About Sleep

The key is to practice. Some of us can naturally bring up sleep and talk about it, other people need checklists and scripts, at least at the beginning. So, don't be afraid to write yourself a checklist and to practice on your team and family until you can do this. It's OK to feel nervous when you start something new, but if you overcome your fear, you will have the power to change your patients' lives.

If You're Having Trouble Finding Patients

Remember, you just need ONE first patient. Once you help one person, word will spread. But don't be afraid to brag about helping people.

Make sleep screening a part of every patient's appointment at least once a year. Their family doctors are most likely not doing this. Their specialists aren't doing this. You may well be the only person on their medical team to ask, "Do you ever fall asleep at the wheel?" Screening saves lives. None of us like to lose a patient – sleep screening is a concrete thing you can do to help your patients get healthier.

You've Got This!

If you're still nervous, take a deep breath, and just get started on treating patients. You've got this. Your training makes you the specialist who is best suited to helping your parents with airway issues. You're going to change and save lives, and you're going to make your practice, and the world, a better place.

Welcome to the world of adult and pediatric airway dentistry. We're glad to have you on our life-saving team.

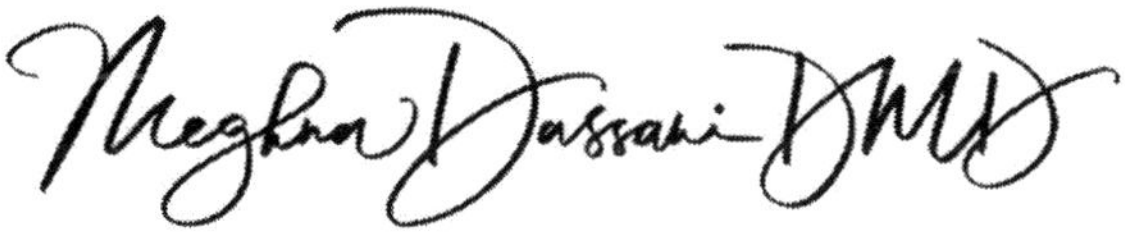

Made in United States
Orlando, FL
04 November 2026

90202572R10103